PHLEBOTOMY
Examination
Review

PHLEBOTOMY
Examination
Review

Kathleen Becan-McBride, EdD, MT (ASCP), CLS(NCA)
Program Director and Professor
Program in Clinical Laboratory Sciences
School of Allied Health Sciences
Associate Professor
Department of Pathology and Laboratory Medicine Medical School
Associate Professor
Graduate School of Biomedical Sciences
UTHSC Valley/Border Coordinator-Health Services Projects

The University of Texas Health Science Center
Texas Medical Center
Houston, Texas

Diana Garza, EdD, MT(ASCP), CLS(NCA)
Associate Professor
Health Care Administration
Texas Woman's University

Clinical Associate Professor
Program in Clinical Laboratory Sciences
The University of Texas Health Science Center
Texas Medical Center
Houston, Texas

APPLETON & LANGE
Norwalk, Connecticut/San Mateo, California

0-8385-7829-2

Copyright © 1991 by Appleton & Lange
A Publishing Division of Prentice Hall

91 92 93 94 95 / 10 9 8 7 6 5 4 3 2 1

Prentice Hall International (UK) Limited, *London*
Prentice Hall of Australia Pty. Limited, *Sydney*
Prentice Hall Canada, Inc., *Toronto*
Prentice Hall Hispanoamericana, S.A., *Mexico*
Prentice Hall of India Private Limited, *New Delhi*
Prentice Hall of Japan, Inc., *Tokyo*
Simon & Schuster Asia Pte. Ltd., *Singapore*
Editora Prentice Hall do Brasil Ltda., *Rio de Janeiro*
Prentice Hall, *Englewood Cliffs, New Jersey*

Library of Congress Cataloging-in-Publication Data

Becan-McBride, Kathleen, 1949–
    Phlebotomy examination review / Kathleen Becan-McBride, Diana Garza.
        p.   cm.
    Sequenced and referenced to be used with: Phlebotomy handbook / Diana Garza, Kathleen Becan-McBride. 2nd. ed. c1989.
    ISBN 0-8385-7829-2
    1. Phlebotomy—Examinations, questions, etc. I. Garza, Diana. II. Garza, Diana. Phlebotomy handbook. III. Title.
    [DNLM: 1. Blood Specimen Collection—examination questions. 2. Bloodletting—examination questions.   QV 39 G245p 1989 Suppl.]
    RB45.15.G37   1989 Suppl.
    616.07'561'076—dc20
    DNLM/DLC
    for Library of Congress   91-4533
                                                                    CIP

Acquisitions Editor: Stephany S. Scott
Production Editor: Sandra K. Huggard
Designer: Steven Byrum
Cover: Michael J. Kelly

PRINTED IN THE UNITED STATES OF AMERICA

Contents

Preface

The dramatic increase in clinical laboratory techniques, automated instruments, and analyses has led to a great demand for proper collection of patient specimens. Thus, the **phlebotomist** is becoming an increasingly important member of the clinical laboratory team. Numerous phlebotomy educational programs have been implemented in order to prepare individuals for the responsibilities of phlebotomists. In addition, national board certifications for phlebotomists have become available.

Due to these important events in phlebotomy, this book has been designed to act as a study companion for students and phlebotomists who are: (1) preparing for national board certification examination(s) and/or (2) pursuing self-assessment in phlebotomy.

The book includes multiple-choice, true-false, fill-in-the-blank, and matching questions as a means to the overall review of phlebotomy. Each chapter in this book is sequenced and referenced to the *Phlebotomy Handbook* (Appleton & Lange, 1989). Thus, after the reader learns the essential topics of phlebotomy in the *Phlebotomy Handbook,* he or she can review these topics through the questions presented in this book. Also, this book may stand alone as a review book since it contains referenced explanatory answers. This edition incorporates illustrations of phlebotomy equipment and techniques as bases for questions to help sharpen phlebotomy skills.

Using this book will assist the reader in identifying areas of relative strength and weakness in the command of phlebotomy skills and responsibilities. It is the intent of this book to serve both the purposes of: (1) preparing students and phlebotomists for taking examinations and (2) helping practicing phlebotomists refresh their knowledge-base in this expanding field of clinical laboratory sciences.

CHAPTER 1

Phlebotomy and the Health Care Setting

Questions

DIRECTIONS: Each of the questions or incomplete statements below is followed by suggested answers or completions. Select the BEST answer in each case.

1. Which of the following statements best describes the role of the phlebotomist in the health care environment?

    (A) starts glucose tolerance procedures and obtains blood specimens by venipuncture or microcollection
    (B) starts IV lines and obtains histologic specimens by appropriate means and facilitates collection and transportation of these specimens
    (C) collects patients' blood by venipuncture or microcollection and facilitates radioisotopic analysis by transporting the specimens to the radiology department
    (D) obtains patients' body fluids by required surgical techniques and facilitates collection and transportation of these specimens

2. The rapid plasma reagin (RPR) test usually is run in which of the following clinical laboratory sections?

    (A) clinical chemistry
    (B) clinical immunology
    (C) clinical microbiology
    (D) hematology

3. Which of the following hospital departments requires the use of heat, cold, water exercise, ultrasound or electricity, and other physical techniques to restore the patient's activity?

    (A) radiology
    (B) occupational therapy

(C) radiation therapy

(D) physical therapy

4. Which of the following is an instrument usually found in the encephalography department?

(A) ECG

(B) EKG

(C) EEG

(D) EGK

5. Of the following personnel, which is sometimes referred to as clinical laboratory technician?

(A) medical technologist

(B) phlebotomist

(C) medical laboratory technician

(D) clinical laboratory scientist

6. Which of the following clinical laboratory sections performs the direct antiglobulin (Coombs) test?

(A) blood bank/transfusion medicine

(B) cytology

(C) histology

(D) clinical microbiology

7. Ionizing radiation for treating disease and fluoroscopic and radiographic x-ray instrumentation are used in what hospital department?

(A) occupational therapy

(B) physical therapy

(C) clinical laboratory

(D) radiology

8. Which of the following best describes the clinical microbiology section?

(A) principal tasks of culturing and identifying bacterial pathogens

(B) major tasks of providing microorganisms to patients

(C) principal tasks of providing blood products to patients

(D) major tasks of providing detailed study of individual chromosomes

9. To become a medical technologist or a clinical laboratory scientist requires which of the following educational degrees as a minimum?

(A) associate's degree

(B) bachelor's degree

(C) master's degree
(D) doctorate degree

10. A primary consultant on drug therapy is a/an

(A) occupational therapist
(B) physical therapist
(C) pharmacist
(D) laboratory supervisor

DIRECTIONS: Each group of lettered words or phrases below is followed by a list of numbered words or phrases. MATCH the lettered word or phrase most closely associated with the numbered word or phrase.

Questions 11 through 15

A.	WBC	**11.** Hemoglobin
B.	Hgb or Hb	**12.** Hematocrit
C.	Hct or Crit	**13.** Differential white count
D.	Diff	**14.** Red blood cell count
E.	RBC	**15.** White blood cell count

DIRECTIONS: For each of the questions or incomplete statements below, ONE or MORE of the numbered responses are correct. In each case, select

A. if only 1, 2, and 3 are correct
B. if only 1 and 3 are correct
C. if only 2 and 4 are correct
D. if only 4 is correct
E. if all are correct

16. The phlebotomist has which of the following duties and responsibilities?

(1) collects blood specimens by venipuncture
(2) collects tissue specimens by catherization
(3) starts glucose tolerance procedures and collects remaining specimens at required times
(4) injects radioactive dyes into the patient and then collects blood specimens by venipuncture or microcollection

17. Which department(s) apply/applies high-energy x-rays, cobalt, and other types of radiation in the treatment of disease, especially cancer?

(1) nuclear medicine
(2) physical therapy

(3) radiology

(4) radiation therapy

18. The medical technologist is sometimes referred to as

    (1) MT

    (2) CLS

    (3) clinical laboratory scientist

    (4) MTL

19. Which of the following is/are examples of health care facilities in which phlebotomists may be employed?

    (1) medical group practice

    (2) HMO

    (3) multiphasic screening center

    (4) neighborhood health center

20. In the clinical chemistry section, the following assay(s) is/are usually performed?

    (1) total proteins

    (2) triglycerides

    (3) cholesterol

    (4) fibrinogen

21. A physician who usually has extensive education in the study and diagnosis of diseases through the use of laboratory test results is sometimes referred to as a/an

    (1) technical supervisor

    (2) administrative technologist

    (3) medical technologist

    (4) pathologist

22. The clinical laboratory department is composed of the following areas

    (1) clinical pharmacy

    (2) clinical pathology

    (3) clinical encephalography

    (4) anatomic pathology

23. Which of the following is/are considered clinical laboratory personnel?

    (1) phlebotomist

    (2) MLT

    (3) MT

    (4) radiologist

DIRECTIONS: Indicate whether each statement is TRUE or FALSE.

24. **True/False:** CBC usually is performed in the hematology area.
25. **True/False:** ABO and $Rh_o(D)$ typing is performed in the blood banking area.
26. **True/False:** Rheumatoid factor (RF) determination usually is performed in the urinalysis area.
27. **True/False:** The platelet count usually is performed in the immunohematology area.
28. **True/False:** The ova and parasites (O & P) test usually is performed in the clinical microbiology laboratory.
29. **True/False:** Serum creatinine determination usually is performed in the clinical chemistry area.
30. **True/False:** Blood urea nitrogen (BUN) usually is determined in the blood banking area.
31. **True/False:** Partial thromboplastin time (PTT) usually is determined in the immunohematology area.
32. **True/False:** The gram stain usually is performed in the clinical microbiology laboratory.
33. **True/False:** (AFB) Acid-Fast bacilli culture is performed in the clinical chemistry area.

DIRECTIONS: Each of the questions or incomplete statements below is followed by suggested answers or completions. Select the BEST answer in each case.

34. Specimens for clinical microbiologic analysis must be handled with extreme care, since they are a

    (A) fire hazard
    (B) radiation hazard
    (C) biohazard
    (D) chemical hazard

35. Which of the following laboratory sections is involved in preparation and processing of tissue samples removed during surgery, autopsy, or other medical procedures?

    (A) clinical immunology
    (B) histology
    (C) blood banking
    (D) clinical microbiology

36. Which of the following best describes a responsibility of technical supervisors of clinical laboratory sections?

    (A) performs various chemical, microscopic, microbiologic, or immunologic tests pertaining to patient care and diagnosis

(B) prepares specimens for reference laboratories

(C) prepares daily work schedules to provide adequate coverage and effective use of personnel

(D) collects adequate and correct blood specimens by venipuncture or microcollection from adults, children, and infants

37. The largest group of nongovernmental hospitals is referred to as

(A) community hospitals

(B) psychiatric hospitals

(C) Veterans Administration hospitals

(D) health maintenance hospitals

38. Which the following descriptions best describes the department of electrocardiography? The department

(A) is composed of clinical pathology and anatomic pathology

(B) records the electric current produced by the contractions of the heart muscle

(C) records the brain waves of the patient

(D) uses radioactive material in the diagnosis and treatment of patients and in the study of the disease process

39. Which of the following laboratory sections usually has a toxicology area?

(A) clinical microbiology

(B) cytogenetics

(C) clinical serology

(D) clinical chemistry

40. A microscopic examination performed to identify the presence or absence of crystals, casts, white blood cells, and red blood cells usually is performed in

(A) hematology

(B) immunohematology

(C) urinalysis

(D) serology

DIRECTIONS: Each group of lettered words or phrases below is followed by a list of numbered words or phrases. MATCH the lettered word or phrase most closely associated with the numbered word or phrase.

Questions 41 through 45

A. chromosomal analysis
B. drug therapy
C. autopsies
D. radioisotopes
E. rehabilitative service

41. Nuclear medicine
42. Anatomic pathology
43. Cytogenetics
44. Physical therapy
45. Pharmacy

DIRECTIONS: For each of the questions or incomplete statements below, ONE or MORE of the numbered responses are correct. In each case select

A. if only 1, 2, and 3 are correct
B. if only 1 and 3 are correct
C. if only 2 and 4 are correct
D. if only 4 is correct
E. if all are correct

46. The organizational structure of a typical clinical laboratory has which of the following laboratory personnel BELOW the administrative technologist on the organizational chart?

    (1) hematology supervisor
    (2) medical technologist
    (3) medical technician
    (4) phlebotomist

47. If the phlebotomist has a request to draw blood from a patient for serum electrolytes, the assays performed in clinical chemistry will include

    (1) sodium
    (2) potassium
    (3) chloride
    (4) fluoride

48. Sometimes, the phlebotomist must draw blood for serum lipids, which include

    (1) bilirubin
    (2) triglycerides
    (3) uric acid
    (4) cholesterol

49. When a C and S test is requested in the clinical microbiology department, this refers to

(1) culturing and identifying bacterial pathogens and inhibition of their growth by an antibiotic
(2) chemical testing and selectivity testing
(3) culture and sensitivity testing
(4) microscopic examination to identify crystals and casts

50. Which of the following term(s) appropriately classify/classifies psychiatric hospitals?

(1) multiphasic screening centers
(2) HMOs
(3) neighborhood health centers
(4) special-care hospitals

51. Which of the following department(s) may inject into a patient dyes and/or radioisotopes that can interfere in laboratory assays?

(1) physical therapy
(2) nuclear medicine
(3) occupational therapy
(4) radiology

DIRECTIONS: Indicate whether each statement is TRUE or FALSE.

52. **True/False:** The RPR test usually is performed in the urinalysis area.
53. **True/False:** Blood glucose usually is determined in the clinical chemistry laboratory.
54. **True/False:** When describing laboratory assays, PT stands for physical therapy.
55. **True/False:** The hematology section is concerned with providing blood products to patients.
56. **True/False:** Cytogenetics usually is the section that screens Pap smears for early diagnosis of malignant diseases of the female genital tract.
57. **True/False:** The lactate dehydrogenase (LH) assay usually is performed in the clinical chemistry area.
58. **True/False:** Hemoglobin assay usually is one of the components of the CBC.
59. **True/False:** The ESR is the same test as the sedimentation rate.
60. **True/False:** The medical technician is above the medical technologist in the organizational structure of a typical clinical laboratory.

DIRECTIONS: Each of the questions or incomplete statements below is followed by suggested answers or completions. Select the BEST answer in each case.

61. If the phlebotomist receives a requisition slip to collect blood from a patient for vitamin assays, these assays could include which of the following?

    (A) magnesium
    (B) acetic acid
    (C) ascorbic acid
    (D) blood urea nitrogen

62. Which of the following descriptions best describes the clinical chemistry section?

    (A) principal tasks of providing blood products to patients
    (B) major tasks of providing detailed study of individual chromosomes
    (C) principal tasks of culturing and identifying bacterial pathogens
    (D) principal tasks include running toxicology and hormone assays

63. Which of the following assays is performed in the immunohematology section?

    (A) chromosomal analysis
    (B) *Proteus OX* agglutinins
    (C) direct Coombs test
    (D) ketones

64. Therapeutic drug monitoring usually is performed in which of the following sections?

    (A) clinical immunology
    (B) clinical chemistry
    (C) clinical microscopy
    (D) clinical microbiology

65. Which of the following departments treats patients having physical or mental disabilities through specific types of exercise or work and collaborates with other health professionals (eg, social workers, nursing staff) to plan a therapeutic program of rehabilitating activities for the patient?

    (A) radiation therapy
    (B) occupational therapy
    (C) radiology
    (D) nuclear medicine

66. Cerebrospinal fluid (CSF), biopsy specimens, and gastric secretions are analyzed in which department?

(A) radiation therapy
(B) radiology
(C) nuclear medicine
(D) clinical laboratory

67. Which of the following best describes a task of the pathologist?

    (A) maintains levels of supplies and reagents commensurate with
        workload
    (B) provides consultation and interpretation on surgical and au-
        topsy tissues
    (C) performs various chemical, microscopic, microbiologic, or immu-
        nologic tests pertaining to patient care and diagnosis
    (D) records and reports test results following laboratory procedures

68. The ova and parasites procedure usually is performed in

    (A) hematology
    (B) clinical microscopy
    (C) clinical microbiology
    (D) serology

**DIRECTIONS: Each group of lettered words or phrases below is followed
by a list of numbered words or phrases. MATCH the lettered word or
phrase most closely associated with the numbered word or phrase.**

Questions 69 through 73

A. thyroxine	69. Electrolyte
B. digoxin	70. Hormone
C. chloride	71. Drug
D. lipid	72. Pco_2
E. blood gas	73. Cholesterol

Answers and Explanations

1. **A.** The phlebotomist collects adequate and correct blood specimens
   by venipuncture or microtechnique on adults, children, and infants.
   In addition, he or she starts glucose tolerance procedures and collects
   remaining specimens at required times.

   Garza D, Becan-McBride K. Phlebotomy Handbook. *E. Norwalk, CT: Appleton &
   Lange; 1989:11.*

2. **B.** The clinical immunology section runs procedures to determine antigen-antibody reactions. The RPR assay is run to test for syphilis. *Garza and Becan-McBride, p 16.*

3. **D.** The role of the physical therapy department is to eliminate the patient's disability or to restore as completely as possible his or her mental or physical abilities. *Garza and Becan-McBride, p 5.*

4. **C.** The encephalography department has the electroencephalograph (EEG) that records brain waves. *Garza and Becan-McBride, p 6.*

5. **C.** The medical laboratory technician (MLT) also is referred to as a clinical laboratory technician (CLT). *Garza and Becan-McBride, p 11.*

6. **A.** The blood banking or transfusion medicine department, sometimes referred to as immunohematology, runs the Coombs test. *Garza and Becan-McBride, p 16.*

7. **D.** The radiology department uses ionizing radiation for treating disease, fluoroscopic and radiographic x-ray instrumentation for diagnosing, and radioactive isotopes for diagnosing and treating. *Garza and Becan-McBride, p 3.*

8. **A.** Microbiology, or the clinical microbiology section, has the principal tasks of culturing and identifying bacterial pathogens. *Garza and Becan-McBride, p 15.*

9. **B.** The medical technologist (MT) has a minimum of a bachelor's degree in a biologic science. *Garza and Becan-McBride, p 10.*

10. **C.** The pharmacist is involved with members of the health care team as a primary consultant on drug therapy. *Garza and Becan-McBride, p 6.*

11. **B.** Hemoglobin is frequently abbreviated as Hgb or Hb on a laboratory test requisition slip. *Garza and Becan-McBride, p 14.*

12. **C.** Hematocrit is referred to as Crit or written as Hct on many laboratory test requisition slips. *Garza and Becan-McBride, p 14.*

13. **D.** Diff is the abbreviated term for differential white blood count. *Garza and Becan-McBride, p 14.*

14. **E.** RBC refers to red blood cell count.
Garza and Becan-McBride, p 14.

15. **A.** WBC is a term frequently used for white blood cell count.
Garza and Becan-McBride, p 14.

16. **B.** The phlebotomist collects blood specimens by venipuncture or microcollection techniques. He or she starts glucose tolerance procedures and collects remaining specimens at required times.
Garza and Becan-McBride, p 11.

17. **D.** The radiation therapy department applies high-energy x-rays, cobalt, elution, and other types of radiation in the treatment of disease, especially cancer.
Garza and Becan-McBride, p 4.

18. **A.** The medical technologist is sometimes referred to as a MT or as a clinical laboratory scientist, abbreviated CLS.
Garza and Becan-McBride, p 10.

19. **E** Health care facilities in which phlebotomists may be employed include Health Maintenance Organizations (HMOs), multiphasic screening centers, neighborhood health centers, and medical group practices.
Garza and Becan-McBride, p 2.

20. **A.** In the clinical chemistry section, total proteins, triglycerides, and cholesterol assays usually are run. The fibrinogen assay usually is performed in the hematology section.
Garza and Becan-McBride, pp 12–13.

21. **D.** The pathologist is a physician who has extensive education in pathology (the study and diagnosis of diseases through the use of laboratory test results).
Garza and Becan-McBride, p 10.

22. **C.** The clinical laboratory department is composed of two major areas, clinical pathology and anatomic pathology.
Garza and Becan-McBride, p 7.

23. **A.** The phlebotomist, medical laboratory technician (MLT), and medical technologist (MT) are all clinical laboratory personnel.
Garza and Becan-McBride, pp 10–11.

24. **TRUE.** The CBC (complete blood count) usually is performed in the hematology area.
Garza and Becan-McBride, p 13.

25. **TRUE.** ABO and $Rh_o(D)$ typing is performed in the blood banking area.
Garza and Becan-McBride, p 13.

26. **FALSE.** Rheumatoid factor (RF) determination usually is performed in the clinical immunology area.
Garza and Becan-McBride, p 13.

27. **FALSE.** The platelet count usually is performed in the hematology or coagulation area.
Garza and Becan-McBride, p 13.

28. **TRUE.** The ova and parasites (O & P) test usually is performed in the clinical microbiology laboratory.
Garza and Becan-McBride, p 13.

29. **TRUE.** Serum creatinine determination usually is performed in the clinical chemistry area.
Garza and Becan-McBride, p 13.

30. **FALSE.** Blood urea nitrogen (BUN) usually is determined in the clinical chemistry area.
Garza and Becan-McBride, p 13.

31. **FALSE.** Partial thromboplastin time (PTT) usually is determined in the hematology or coagulation area.
Garza and Becan-McBride, p 13.

32. **TRUE.** The gram stain usually is performed in the clinical microbiology laboratory.
Garza and Becan-McBride, p 13.

33. **FALSE.** AFB culture is performed in the clinical microbiology laboratory.
Garza and Becan-McBride, p 13.

34. **C.** Specimens for microbiologic analysis may be highly infectious and, thus, are considered biohazardous.
Garza and Becan-McBride, p 16.

35. **B.** The histology section is involved in the preparation and processing of tissue samples removed during surgery, autopsy, or other medical procedures.
Garza and Becan-McBride, p 17.

36. **C.** One of the many responsibilities of the technical supervisor of clinical laboratory sections is to prepare daily schedules to provide adequate coverage and effective use of personnel.
Garza and Becan-McBride, p 10.

37. **A.** The largest group of nongovernmental hospitals is referred to as community hospitals.
     Garza and Becan-McBride, p 2.

38. **B.** The department of electrocardiography is used as a diagnostic service to record the electric current produced by the contractions of the heart muscle.
     Garza and Becan-McBride, p 6.

39. **D.** The clinical chemistry section usually has a toxicology area for drug analysis.
     Garza and Becan-McBride, p 12.

40. **C.** A microscopic examination performed to identify the presence or absence of crystals, casts, white blood cells, and red blood cells usually is performed in urinalysis.
     Garza and Becan-McBride, p 15.

41. **D.** Nuclear medicine uses radioisotopes in the diagnosis and treatment of patients.
     Garza and Becan-McBride, p 4.

42. **C.** Anatomic pathology is involved in the performance of autopsies.
     Garza and Becan-McBride, p 7.

43. **A.** Cytogenetic techniques provide detailed study of individual chromosomes.
     Garza and Becan-McBride, p 17.

44. **E.** The physical therapy department provides rehabilitative service to patients.
     Garza and Becan-McBride, p 5.

45. **B.** The pharmacy department provides consultation on drug therapy for patients.
     Garza and Becan-McBride, p 6.

46. **E.** The administrative technologist oversees the activities of the hematology supervisor, medical technologist, medical technician, and phlebotomist. Thus, they are all below the administrative technologist on the organizational chart.
     Garza and Becan-McBride, p 8.

47. **A.** Blood drawn for an electrolyte panel usually includes testing for sodium, potassium, bicarbonate, and chloride.
     Garza and Becan-McBride, p 12.

48. **C.** Serum lipids are the triglyceride and cholesterol assays performed usually in the clinical chemistry area.
     Garza and Becan-McBride, p 12.

49. **B.** A "C and S" test is a culture and sensitivity test performed in clinical microbiology. This test involves culturing and identifying bacterial pathogens and testing for inhibition of bacterial growth by an antibiotic.
Garza and Becan-McBride, p 15.

50. **D.** Psychiatric hospitals are special-care hospitals, since they treat only a few types of illnesses.
Garza and Becan-McBride, p 2.

51. **C.** Radiology studies sometimes require that the patient be injected with dye. Radioisotopes are injected intravenously into patients in the nuclear medicine department for diagnostic and treatment purposes.
Garza and Becan-McBride, p 4.

52. **FALSE.** The RPR test usually is performed in the clinical immunology/serology laboratory section.
Garza and Becan-McBride, p 13.

53. **TRUE.** Blood glucose determination usually is performed in the clinical chemistry laboratory section.
Garza and Becan-McBride, p 12.

54. **FALSE.** PT in the laboratory refers to prothrombin time.
Garza and Becan-McBride, p 14.

55. **FALSE.** The immunohematology (blood banking) section has the major tasks of providing blood products to patients.
Garza and Becan-McBride, p 16.

56. **FALSE.** The section of cytogenetics provides chromosomal analysis, whereas the cytology section screens Pap smears.
Garza and Becan-McBride, pp 16–17.

57. **TRUE.** Lactate dehydrogenase (LH) is an enzyme assay performed in the clinical chemistry area.
Garza and Becan-McBride, p 12.

58. **TRUE.** One of the components of the complete blood count (CBC) is the hemoglobin assay.
Garza and Becan-McBride, p 14.

59. **TRUE.** ESR stands for erythrocyte sedimentation rate, which is referred to also as the sedimentation rate.
Garza and Becan-McBride, p 14.

60. **FALSE.** The medical technologist is above the medical technician is the organizational structure of a typical clinical laboratory.
Garza and Becan-McBride, pp 8–9.

61. **C.** A vitamin assay that is sometimes run on a patient is ascorbic acid (vitamin C).
    Garza and Becan-McBride, p 12.

62. **D.** Principal tasks of the clinical chemistry section include running toxicology and hormone assays.
    Garza and Becan-McBride, p 12.

63. **C.** The direct Coombs test is performed in the immunohematology section.
    Garza and Becan-McBride, p 13.

64. **B.** The clinical chemistry section usually performs therapeutic drug monitoring.
    Garza and Becan-McBride, p 12.

65. **B.** The occupational therapist treats patients having physical or mental disabilities through specific types of exercise or work and collaborates with other health professionals (eg, social workers, nursing staff, attending physician, physical therapist) to plan a therapeutic program of rehabilitating activities for the patient.
    Garza and Becan-McBride, p 5.

66. **D.** The clinical laboratory department analyzes various body fluids and tissues, including cerebrospinal fluid (CSF), biopsy specimens, and gastric secretions.
    Garza and Becan-McBride, p 7.

67. **B.** A major task of the pathologist is to provide consultation and interpretation on surgical and autopsy tissues.
    Garza and Becan-McBride, p 10.

68. **C.** The ova and parasites procedure usually is performed in the clinical microbiology section.
    Garza and Becan-McBride, p 13.

69. **C.** Chloride is an electrolyte.
    Garza and Becan-McBride, p 12.

70. **A.** Thyroxine is a hormone.
    Garza and Becan-McBride, p 12.

71. **B.** Digoxin is a medication, sometimes referred to as a drug.
    Garza and Becan-McBride, p 12.

72. **E.** Pco_2 is part of the blood gas analysis.
    Garza and Becan-McBride, p 12.

73. **D.** Cholesterol is one of the main lipids tested for in the clinical laboratory.
    Garza and Becan-McBride, p 12.

CHAPTER 2

Anatomy and Physiology of Body Systems

Questions

DIRECTIONS: Each group of lettered words or phrases below is followed by a list of numbered words or phrases. MATCH the lettered word or phrase most closely associated with the numbered word or phrase.

Questions 1 through 4

A. anabolism
B. catabolism
C. homeostasis
D. metabolism

1. Maintaining a steady state in the body
2. Breaking down substances to use energy
3. Chemical reaction in cells to change complex substances into simpler ones while producing energy
4. Cells use energy to make complex compounds from simple ones

Questions 5 through 13

A. skeletal system
B. digestive system
C. muscular system
D. circulatory system
E. urinary system
F. nervous system
G. respiratory system
H. endocrine system
I. reproductive system

5. Neurons, brain, spinal cord
6. Kidneys, ureters, bladder, urethra
7. Bones and joints
8. Glands that release hormones
9. Ovulation, fertilization, menstruation
10. Skeletal, visceral, striated muscles
11. Exchange of gases between air and blood
12. Transports blood cells, water, and other constituents
13. Breaks down food chemically for absorption

Questions 14 through 18 (May have more than 1 answer in this section)

A. oxyhemoglobin
B. carboxyhemoglobin
C. lung capillaries
D. alveoli
E. larynx

14. Hemoglobin plus oxygen
15. Voice box
16. Sacs in the lungs that allow diffusion between air and blood.
17. Hemoglobin plus carbon dioxide
18. Where dissociation of oxygen and hemoglobin takes place

Questions 19 through 24 (May have more than one answer in this section)

A. red blood cells
B. white blood cells
C. platelets
D. plasma
E. serum
F. granulocytes

19. Leukocytes
20. Erythrocytes
21. Thrombocytes
22. Basophils
23. Blood containing anticoagulant
24. Blood without anticoagulant

Questions 25 through 27

A. capillaries
B. arteries
C. veins

25. Carry deoxygenated blood toward the heart
26. Carry oxygenated blood away from the heart
27. Microscopic vessels that link arterioles and venules

Questions 28 through 33

A. radial vein
B. brachial vein
C. great saphenous vein
D. tibial vein
E. jugular vein
F. vena cava
G. hepatic vein
H. renal vein

28. Neck
29. Heart
30. Liver
31. Arm
32. Leg
33. Kidney

Questions 34 through 41

A. thrombocyte
B. erythrocyte

34. Normal range, 5000 to 9000/mm^3
35. Normal range, 250,000 to 450,000/mm^3

C. leukocyte

D. reticulocyte

E. myelocyte

F. megakaryocyte

G. stem cell

H. monoblast

36. Normal range, 4.5 to 5.5 million/mm^3

37. An immature red blood cell

38. Undifferentiated immature blood cell

39. An immature granulocyte

40. An immature platelet

41. An immature monocyte

DIRECTIONS: Each of the questions or incomplete statements below is followed by suggested answers or completions. Select the BEST answer in each case.

42. Meninges are defined as

   (A) the causative agent of meningitis

   (B) protective membrane coverings of the brain and spinal cord

   (C) nerve impulses that transmit sensory functions

   (D) cranial nerves

43. Which organ secretes bile?

   (A) pancreas

   (B) stomach

   (C) appendix

   (D) liver

44. Glomeruli are best described as

   (A) filters of the kidney

   (B) cells in the liver

   (C) part of the digestive system

   (D) part of the endocrine system

45. The endocrine system can best be evaluated by

   (A) tissue biopsy

   (B) analyzing hormone levels

   (C) doing blood gas analyses

   (D) testing spinal fluid

46. Leukocytes function primarily as

   (A) oxygen transport mechanisms

   (B) host cells

   (C) clotting mechanisms

   (D) defense mechanisms

47. Erythrocytes function primarily as

   (A) oxygen transport mechanisms

   (B) host cells

(C) clotting mechanisms

(D) defense mechanisms

48. Platelets function primarily as

(A) oxygen transport mechanisms

(B) host cells

(C) clotting mechanisms

(D) defense mechanisms

DIRECTIONS: For each of the questions or incomplete statements below, ONE or MORE of the numbered responses are correct. In each case select

A. if only 1, 2, and 3 are correct

B. if only 1 and 3 are correct

C. if only 2 and 4 are correct

D. if only 4 is correct

E. if all are correct

49. The skeletal system serves the body in which way(s)?

(1) support and protection

(2) movement and leverage

(3) hematopoiesis

(4) calcium storage

50. Laboratory tests that evaluate the skeletal system are

(1) serum calcium

(2) alkaline phosphatase

(3) synovial fluid analysis

(4) urine culture

51. The nervous system is composed of which component(s)?

(1) brain

(2) spinal fluid

(3) spinal cord

(4) meninges

52. If a blood specimen is allowed to clot (without anticoagulant), what remains?

(1) fibrin clot

(2) blood cells

(3) serum

(4) plasma

53. Plasma has which of the following features?

    (1) contains anticoagulants
    (2) contains approximately 90% water
    (3) can be separated by centrifugation
    (4) is the liquid portion of the blood

54. The human heart has which of the following features?

    (1) is the size of a man's fist
    (2) has four chambers
    (3) is located slightly left of the midline
    (4) is a gland

55. Capillaries have which of the following features?

    (1) may be so small that only one cell can pass through
    (2) have sensitive nerve endings
    (3) link arterioles to venules
    (4) are located only in the fingers

56. Tests for blood types usually are performed in which laboratory(ies)?

    (1) virology
    (2) bacteriology
    (3) chemistry
    (4) blood bank/transfusion medicine

57. Meningitis can be detected by which of the following methods?

    (1) blood analyses
    (2) urine cultures
    (3) measuring carbon dioxide
    (4) spinal fluid cultures

58. Components of the respiratory system include which of the following?

    (1) nose
    (2) trachea
    (3) lungs
    (4) humerus

59. Red blood cells have which of the following features?

    (1) measure about 7 μm in diameter
    (2) normally have no nucleus in circulating blood
    (3) carry oxygen and carbon dioxide
    (4) have a biconcave disc shape

60. Red blood cells contain

(1) hemoglobin
(2) granules
(3) blood type antigens on the surface membrane
(4) bile

Answers

1. **C.**

   Garza D, Becan-McBride K. Phlebotomy Handbook. E. Norwalk, CT: Appleton & Lange; 1989:22–23.

2. **D.**

   Garza and Becan-McBride, pp 22–23.

3. **B.**

   Garza and Becan-McBride, pp 22–23.

4. **A.**

   Garza and Becan-McBride, pp 22–23.

5. **F.**

   Garza and Becan-McBride, pp 24–37.

6. **E.**

   Garza and Becan-McBride, pp 24–37.

7. **A.**

   Garza and Becan-McBride, pp 24–37.

8. **H.**

   Garza and Becan-McBride, pp 24–37.

9. **I.**

   Garza and Becan-McBride, pp 24–37.

10. **C.**

    Garza and Becan-McBride, pp 24–37.

11. **G.**

    Garza and Becan-McBride, pp 24–37.

12. **D.**

    Garza and Becan-McBride, pp 24–37.

13. **B.**

    Garza and Becan-McBride, pp 24–37.

14. **A.**
Garza and Becan-McBride, p 27.

15. **E.**
Garza and Becan-McBride, p 27.

16. **B.**
Garza and Becan-McBride, p 27.

17. **B.**
Garza and Becan-McBride, p 27.

18. **C, D.**
Garza and Becan-McBride, p 27.

19. **B, F.**
Garza and Becan-McBride, pp 29–37.

20. **A.**
Garza and Becan-McBride, pp 29–37.

21. **C.**
Garza and Becan-McBride, pp 29–37.

22. **B, F.**
Garza and Becan-McBride, pp 29–37.

23. **D.**
Garza and Becan-McBride, pp 29–37.

24. **E.**
Garza and Becan-McBride, pp 29–37.

25. **C.**
Garza and Becan-McBride, pp 27.

26. **B.**
Garza and Becan-McBride, p 27.

27. **A.**
Garza and Becan-McBride, p 27.

28. **E.**
Garza and Becan-McBride, pp 37–38.

29. **F.**
Garza and Becan-McBride, pp 37–38.

30. **G.**
Garza and Becan-McBride, pp 37–38.

31. **A, B.**
    Garza and Becan-McBride, pp 37–38.

32. **C, D.**
    Garza and Becan-McBride, pp 37–38.

33. **H.**
    Garza and Becan-McBride, pp 37–38.

34. **C.**
    Garza and Becan-McBride, pp 32–34.

35. **A.**
    Garza and Becan-McBride, pp 32–34.

36. **B.**
    Garza and Becan-McBride, pp 32–34.

37. **D.**
    Garza and Becan-McBride, pp 32–34.

38. **G.**
    Garza and Becan-McBride, pp 32–34.

39. **E.**
    Garza and Becan-McBride, pp 32–34.

40. **F.**
    Garza and Becan-McBride, pp 32–34.

41. **H.**
    Garza and Becan-McBride, pp 32–34.

42. **B.**
    Garza and Becan-McBride, p 26.

43. **D.**
    Garza and Becan-McBride, p 28.

44. **A.**
    Garza and Becan-McBride, p 28.

45. **B.**
    Garza and Becan-McBride, p 29.

46. **D.**
    Garza and Becan-McBride, p 34.

47. **A.**
    Garza and Becan-McBride, p 30.

48. **C.**

    Garza and Becan-McBride, p 34.

49. **E.**

    Garza and Becan-McBride, pp 24–25.

50. **A.**

    Garza and Becan-McBride, pp 24–25.

51. **E.**

    Garza and Becan-McBride, p 26.

52. **A.**

    Garza and Becan-McBride, p 35.

53. **E.**

    Garza and Becan-McBride, pp 34–35.

54. **A.**

    Garza and Becan-McBride, pp 35–36.

55. **B.**

    Garza and Becan-McBride, pp 37–38.

56. **D.**

    Garza and Becan-McBride, p 33.

57. **D.**

    Garza and Becan-McBride, p 26.

58. **A.**

    Garza and Becan-McBride, p 27.

59. **E.**

    Garza and Becan-McBride, p 30.

60. **B.**

    Garza and Becan-McBride, p 30.

CHAPTER 3

Collection Reagents, Supplies, and Interfering Chemical Substances

Questions

DIRECTIONS: Each of the questions or incomplete statements below is followed by suggested answers or completions. Select the BEST answer in each case.

1. Which of the following anticoagulants is found in a blue-stoppered blood collecting vacuum tube?

    (A) EDTA
    (B) sodium heparin
    (C) sodium citrate
    (D) ammonium oxalate

2. Blood gases are collected with which of the following anticoagulants?

    (A) EDTA
    (B) heparin
    (C) oxalate
    (D) citrate

3. Which of the following has been introduced to help in the prevention of accidental needlesticks?

    (A) HR needle* (ICU Medical, Inc., Mission Viejo, CA)
    (B) Monoject Corvac tube (Monoject Scientific, a Division of Sherwood Medical, St. Louis, MO)
    (C) Microtainer (Becton-Dickinson and Co., Rutherford, NJ)
    (D) Autolet (Ulster Scientific, Inc., Highland, NY)

4. If a blood specimen is allowed to clot, the result is

    (A) plasma plus blood cells
    (B) serum plus blood cells

(C) anticoagulated blood

(D) serum plus plasma

5. Which of the following is obtained through a lumbar puncture?

(A) pleural fluid

(B) cerebrospinal fluid

(C) synovial fluid

(D) peritoneal fluid

DIRECTIONS: Each group of lettered words or phrases below is followed by a list of numbered words or phrases. MATCH the lettered word or phrase most closely associated with the numbered word or phrase.

Questions 6 through 10

A. inhibition of the chromogenic or fluorescent reaction

B. CAP

C. pancreatitis

D. drug-induced hepatotoxicity

E. elevation of blood urea nitrogen (BUN)

6. Elevation of serum amylase

7. Elevation of alanine aminotransferase

8. Medication leading to renal impairment

9. College of American Pathologists

10. Falsely decreased value of the blood analyte

Questions 11 through 15

A. lithium heparin

B. EDTA

C. inert polymer barrier

D. potassium oxalate and sodium fluoride

E. sodium heparin

11. Lavender-stoppered tube

12. Gray-stoppered tube

13. Green-stoppered tube

14. Royal blue-stoppered tube

15. Gray and red-stoppered tube

DIRECTIONS: Indicate whether each statement is TRUE or FALSE.

16. **True/False:** Sterile blood specimens are not always required for blood cultures.

17. **True/False:** As shown in Figure 3–1, the phlebotomy resheather system decreases the possibility of accidental needlesticks and, thus, transmission of AIDS and other infectious diseases to phlebotomists.

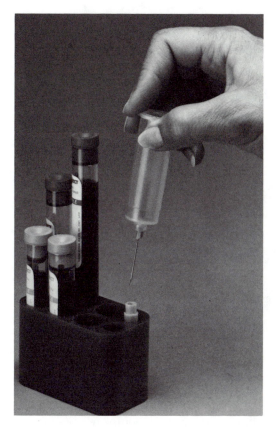

Figure 3–1. *(Courtesy of Datar Inc., Long Lake, MN.)*

18. **True/False:** The gauge number indicates the diameter of the needle, and the larger the number, the larger the needle.

19. **True/False:** EDTA is the same anticoagulant as ethylenediaminetetraacetate.

20. **True/False:** The B-D Safety-Lok needle holder, as shown in Figure 3–2, is used to lock a blood collection vacuum tube into a holder so that the vacuum tube will not move.

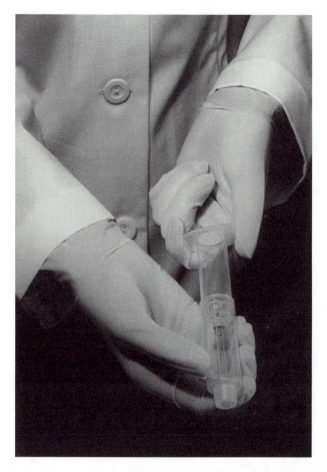

Figure 3–2. B-D Vacutainer Safety-Lok needle holder. *(Courtesy of Becton Dickinson Vacutainer Systems, Rutherford, NJ.)*

21. **True/False:** Mainstream urine specimens commonly are used for routine admission urinalysis.
22. **True/False:** Pleural fluid is obtained from the lung cavity.
23. **True/False:** Even though body fluids, such as pleural fluid, are not biohazardous, the phlebotomist should be careful in the transportation of body fluids because they are difficult to obtain.
24. **True/False:** Drug interference leading to falsely decreased results in blood specimens may be caused by the drug competing with the chromogenic reagent for peroxide in a peroxide-generating reaction, thus falsely decreasing the chromogen oxidation and concentration of the blood analyte.

DIRECTIONS: For each of the questions or incomplete statements below, ONE or MORE of the numbered responses are correct. In each case select

A. if only 1, 2, and 3 are correct
B. if only 1 and 3 are correct
C. if only 2 and 4 are correct
D. if only 4 is correct
E. if all are correct

25. Which of the following item(s) is/are typically carried on a microcollection tray?

    (1) heparinized Natelson tubes, 75 μL
    (2) disposable gloves
    (3) lancets
    (4) alcohol or Betadine pads

26. Which of the following is/are good reasons to perform a capillary blood collection on an adult?

    (1) severely burned patient
    (2) veins that are difficult to stick because of their small size or location
    (3) extreme obesity
    (4) thrombotic tendencies

27. Which of the following is/are capillary blood collection system(s)?

    (1) Microvette
    (2) Unopette
    (3) Microtainer
    (4) microtome

28. Which of the following is/are tourniquet(s) used in venipuncture?

    (1) Penrose
    (2) strap
    (3) rubber hose
    (4) blood pressure cuff

29. Which of the following anticoagulant(s) is/are used frequently in coagulation blood studies?

    (1) citrate phosphate dextrose
    (2) sodium citrate
    (3) acid citrate dextrose
    (4) sodium oxalate

30. Which of the following anticoagulant(s) is/are used frequently in clinical cytogenetic studies?

    (1) sodium citrate
    (2) sodium oxalate
    (3) ammonium oxalate
    (4) sodium heparin

31. Which of the following is/are fluids that the phlebotomists may be involved in transporting to the laboratory for the necessary analyses?

    (1) gastric secretions
    (2) peritoneal fluid
    (3) pleural fluid
    (4) CSF

DIRECTIONS: Each group of lettered words or phrases below is followed by a list of numbered words or phrases. MATCH the lettered word or phrase most closely associated with the numbered word or phrase.

Questions 32 through 36

A. whole blood (purple-stoppered blood collection tube)
B. serum (red-stoppered blood collection tube)
C. whole blood (green-stoppered blood collection tube)
D. plasma (blue-stoppered blood collection tube)
E. plasma (gray-stoppered blood collection tube)

32. Chromosome analysis
33. Blood cell count (WBC, RBC, Hgb, Hct, MCV, MCH, MCHC)
34. Alkaline phosphatase
35. Fasting blood glucose
36. Antithrombin III

Questions 37 through 41

A. B-D Unopette
B. heparinized Natelson tubes, 75 μL
C. butterfly

37. A commonly used intravenous device
38. Used frequently in the micro-collection of blood gases

D Corvac tube

E B-D Microtainer without anti-coagulant

39. Serum separation tube

40. Used frequently to collect electro-lytes and general chemistry micro-specimens

41. Prefilled device used as a collec-tion and dilution unit

DIRECTIONS: Each of the questions or incomplete statements below is followed by suggested answers or completetions. Select the BEST answer in each case.

42. Tylenol (acetaminophen) can lead to which of the following errors in laboratory results?

(A) falsely increased values in skeletal muscle enzyme assays
(B) falsely increased values in liver function tests
(C) falsely decreased values in liver function tests
(D) falsely decreased values in skeletal muscle enzyme assays

43. Falsely decreased laboratory results for the blood analyte can be

(A) mistakenly interpreted as normal when the blood analyte is truly in the subnormal range
(B) caused by increasing the color produced in the laboratory assay
(C) mistakenly interpreted as normal or subnormal if the blood analyte is truly in an elevated range or normal range, respec-tively
(D) caused by a medication competing with the blood analyte for a chromogenic reagent, thus falsely decreasing the resultant color of the reaction

44. A blood collection vacuum tube is part of the

(A) B-D Microtainer system
(B) B-D Vacutainer system
(C) B-D Unopette system
(D) Microvette system

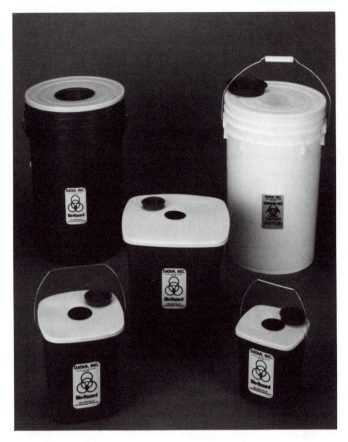

Figure 3–3. *(Courtesy of Datar Inc. Long Lake, MN.)*

45. As shown in Figure 3–3, these containers have been manufactured to be used for

(A) Vacutainer tubes
(B) tourniquets
(C) needles
(D) Corvac tubes

46. Which of the following devices has been developed specifically for the bleeding time assay?

(A) Surgicutt
(B) Autolet
(C) Microvette
(D) Unopette

47. It is recommended to avoid using gloves with talc powder when collecting blood because the tubes of patients' blood may become contaminated with this powder, leading to falsely

(A) decreased iron values
(B) elevated iron values
(C) elevated copper values
(D) elevated calcium values

48. Which of the following blood analytes usually is collected in a red-stoppered blood collection vacuum tube?

(A) WBC count
(B) chromosome analysis
(C) RBC count
(D) alkaline phosphatase

49. Which of the following test procedures usually requires a purple-stoppered blood collection vacuum tube?

(A) serum protein electrophoresis
(B) hematocrit
(C) aldolase
(D) leucine aminopeptidase

50. Which of the following test procedures requires whole blood collected in a purple-stoppered blood collection vacuum tube?

(A) sedimentation rate
(B) thrombin time
(C) kanamycin
(D) lipase

51. Which of the following tests usually requires blood collected in a dark blue-stoppered blood collection vacuum tube?

(A) cortisol
(B) CBC
(C) lactate dehydrogenase
(D) lead

52. In pediatric collections using disposable sterile lancets, such as the Monolet in Figure 3–4, the tip of the lancet is less than how many millimeters in length to avoid penetrating the bone in a newborn's heel?

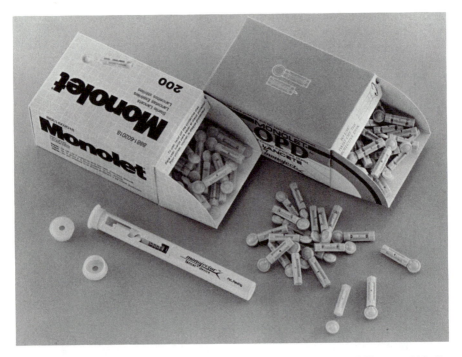

Figure 3—4. Monolet and Monojector lancet device. *(Courtesy of Sherwood Medical, St. Louis, MO.)*

    (A) 2.4 mm
✓ (B) 2.5 mm
    (C) 2.6 mm
    (D) 2.7 mm

53. Falsely increased laboratory results for the blood analyte can be

    (A) caused by a medication competing with the blood analyte for a chromogenic reagent, thus falsely decreasing the resultant color of the reaction

    (B) mistakenly interpreted as elevated or normal if the blood analyte is truly in a normal range or decreased range, respectively

    (C) mistakenly interpreted as normal or subnormal if the blood analyte is truly in an elevated range or normal range, respectively

    (D) caused by decreasing the fluorescence produced in the laboratory assay

DIRECTIONS: Indicate whether each statement is TRUE or FALSE.

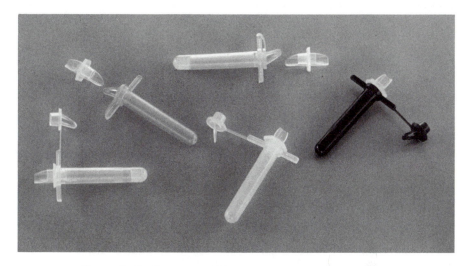

Figure 3—5. *(Courtesy of Sherwood Medical, St. Louis, MO.)*

54. **True/False:** Figure 3–5 is referred to as a Unopette.
55. **True/False:** The Autolet (Ulster Scientific, Inc., Highland, NY) is a spring-activated puncture device with two disposable platforms for control of penetration depth.
56. **True/False:** During blood collection, if the patient mentions to the phlebotomist that he or she had taken numerous aspirin over the past 2 days for a bad headache, the phlebotomist should call the patient's physician immediately.
57. **True/False:** Blood collection vacuum tubes usually contain silicon to decrease the possibility of hemolysis and prevent the clot from adhering to the wall of the tube.
58. **True/False:** Aerotrap (Innovative Laboratory Products, Ltd., distributed by Fisher Scientific) is used in laboratories to push the blood collection vacuum stopper into the tube after blood is removed.
59. **True/False:** Sterile vacuum collecting tubes are used frequently for trace element studies.
60. **True/False:** Citrate phosphate dextrose (CPD) is an anticoagulant used in collection of blood for blood donations.
61. **True/False:** Sputum is a term used to describe fluid from a wound in the stomach that contains pus.
62. **True/False:** Serum is obtained from whole blood that is mixed with an anticoagulant.
63. **True/False:** Heparin is a mucopolysaccharide used in assays, for example, for ammonia and plasma hemoglobin.

DIRECTIONS: Each group of lettered words or phrases below is followed by a list of numbered words or phrases. MATCH the lettered word or phrase most closely associated with the numbered word or phrase.

Questions 64 through 68

A. erythrocyte fragility test
B. total estrogens
C. bleeding time
D. renin activity
E. leukocyte alkaline phosphatase stain

64. Hemalet
65. Serum collected in a red-stoppered vacuum tube
66. Whole blood collected in a purple-stoppered vacuum tube
67. Six fresh blood smears
68. Whole blood collected in a purple-stoppered vacuum tube and transported in ice

Questions 69 through 73

A. SGPT
B. ESR
C. APTT
D. SGOT
E. PNH

69. Aspartate aminotransferase
70. Sucrose presumptive test
71. Alanine aminotransferase
72. Activated thromboplastin time
73. Sedimentation rate

DIRECTIONS: For each of the questions or incomplete statements below, ONE or MORE of the numbered responses are correct. In each case select

A. if only 1, 2, and 3 are correct
B. if only 1 and 3 are correct
C. if only 2 and 4 are correct
D. if only 4 is correct
E. if all are correct

74. Which of the following is/are frequently collected in a gray-stoppered blood collection vacuum tube?

(1) fasting blood glucose
(2) glucose
(3) FBS
(4) glucose 6-phosphate dehydrogenase

75. Which of the following usually must be collected in sterile vacuum collection tubes?

(1) PT
(2) ESR

(3) trace element studies

(4) activated clotting time

76. Which of the following blood analytes is/are sensitive to light?

(1) lead

(2) glucose

(3) calcium

(4) bilirubin

77. Which of the following proteins is/are found in plasma but not found in serum?

(1) albumin

(2) fibrin

(3) globulins

(4) fibrinogen

78. The platelet function profile needs which of the following specimen type(s) and stopper color(s)?

(1) whole blood (purple)

(2) plasma (blue)

(3) whole blood (blue)

(4) serum (red)

79. Which of the following must be collected in a blue-stoppered blood collection tube?

(1) RVV

(2) Russell viper venom time

(3) Stypven time

(4) VDRL

80. Which of the following is/are blood test(s) for syphilis?

(1)) RPR

(2) TSH

(3) VDRL

(4) ALT

81. Which of the following is/are assays to test specifically for thyroid functioning?

(1) TSH

(2) T$_4$

(3) thyroxine

(4) thrombin time

82. Which of the following would not typically be found on a microcollection tray?

    (1) disposable gloves
    (2) marking pens
    (3) lancets
    (4) needles for vacuum tubes and syringes

DIRECTIONS: Indicate whether each statement is TRUE or FALSE.

83. **True/False:** Figure 3–6 is a photograph of a Unopette.

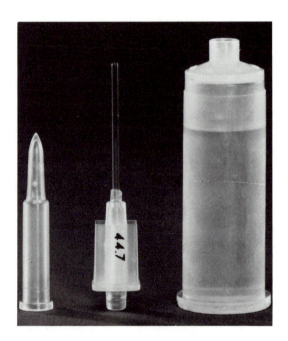

Figure 3–6. *(Courtesy of Becton-Dickinson and Co., Rutherford, NJ.)*

84. **True/False:** If the phlebotomist has the responsibility to receive and sign in 24-hour urine specimens from patients for laboratory assays, it is acceptable protocol for a patient to submit the 24-hour urine specimen in the patient's own jar.

85. **True/False:** For collection of a 24-hour urine specimen, the patient should be instructed to begin the collection process between 1 and 3 PM.

86. **True/False:** Pericardial fluid is obtained from the heart cavity.
87. **True/False:** The fluorescent treponemal antibody test is also referred to as MHA-TP.
88. **True/False:** The low-density lipoproteins assay sometimes is abbreviated on the test requisition slip as LL.
89. **True/False:** The Valium assay is the same test as the diazepam test.
90. **True/False:** HAA is an abbreviation for the hemoglobin A assay.
91. **True/False:** PAS for glycogen is a special stain procedure and requires a blood smear.
92. **True/False:** The laboratory test Monospot is the same as the heterophil antibody test and requires serum collected in a red-stoppered blood collection tube.
93. **True/False:** If the phlebotomist had to collect blood for a Dilantin assay, the blood specimen could be used for the phenytoin assay, since Dilantin and phenytoin are the same.

DIRECTIONS: Each group of lettered words or phrases below is followed by a list of numbered words or phrases. MATCH the lettered word or phrase most closely associated with the numbered word or phrase.

Questions 94 through 98

A. thiamine
B. urea nitrogen
C. thrombin time
D. sucrose presumptive (PNH)
E. vitamin D (25-OH)

94. Whole blood (purple)
95. BUN
96. Whole blood (green)
97. Plasma (blue)
98. Whole blood (blue)

Questions 99 through 103

A. insulin test
B. bilirubin assay
C. glucose
D. microbiology blood specimens
E. Heinz bodies special stain

99. Glycolytic action of the blood cells can interfere in the analysis of this analyte
100. Must be transferred to culture media as quickly as possible
101. Must place tube of blood in ice container immediately after collection
102. Requires a blood smear
103. Blood must be protected from light

Questions 104 through 108

A. whole blood (red)   104. Rosette
B. plasma (blue)   105. Renin activity
C. whole blood (purple)   106. Ferritin
D. plasma (purple)   107. Coombs test
E. serum (red)   108. Factor assay

DIRECTIONS: For each of the questions or incomplete statements below, ONE or MORE of the numbered responses are correct. In each case select

A. if only 1, 2, and 3 are correct
B. if only 1 and 3 are correct
C. if only 2 and 4 are correct
D. if only 4 is correct
E. if all are correct

109. Which of the following statements apply to the B-D Unopette?

   (1) a plastic reservoir containing a premeasured volume of reagent for diluting
   (2) a reusable, self-filling diluting pipette
   (3) consists of a straight, thin-wall, uniform-bore glass capillary tube fitted into a plastic holder
   (4) consists of an automatic blade retraction mechanism

110. For which of the following assays should serum be obtained in a red stopper collection tube?

   (1) zinc
   (2) transaminase
   (3) testosterone
   (4) rubella

111. Gray-stoppered blood collection tubes can be ordered containing

   (1) potassium oxalate and sodium fluoride
   (2) sodium fluoride and thymol
   (3) potassium oxalate
   (4) heparin

112. Which of the following laboratory procedures require(s) a blood smear?

   (1) blood cell count, differential
   (2) carcinoembryonic antigen (CEA)

(3) Heinz bodies special stain
(4) chloramphenicol

113. The A/G ratio refers to which of the following proteins?

(1) alpha-fibrinogen
(2) albumin
(3) gamma-transpeptidase
(4) globulin

114. When the phlebotomist collects blood in a red-stoppered vacuum tube for glucose determination, the serum must be separated from the blood cells within 30 minutes to avoid

(1) hemolysis
(2) glycogenesis
(3) hemoconcentration
(4) glycolysis

115. For which of the following assays must blood be collected in a green-stoppered blood collection tube?

(1) ammonia
(2) chromosome analysis
(3) cryofibrinogen
(4) LE cell test

116. Which of the following is/are true concerning the volume of plasma or serum that generally can be collected from a patient?

(1) 100 to 150 μL of plasma or serum usually can be collected from a premature infant
(2) 200 to 300 μL of plasma or serum usually can be collected from a full-term newborn
(3) larger volumes than 300 μL of plasma or serum usually can be collected from an adult
(4) only 300 μL of plasma or serum usually can be collected from a child

DIRECTIONS: Each of the questions or incomplete statements below is followed by suggested answers or completions. Select the BEST answer in each case.

117. Lancets with which of the following maximum lengths are suitable for older children?

(A) 5 mm maximum length
(B) 6 mm maximum length

(C) 7 mm maximum length
(D) 8 mm maximum length

118. Which of the following is true?

(A) the blood cells are contained in the fibrinogen clot
(B) the serum contains clotting elements
(C) the blood cells are contained in the fibrin clot
(D) the serum contains fibrinogen

119. The tubes shown in Figure 3–7 are used in the collection of

(A) microscopy specimens
(B) clinical chemistry specimens
(C) clinical immunology specimens
(D) microbiology specimens

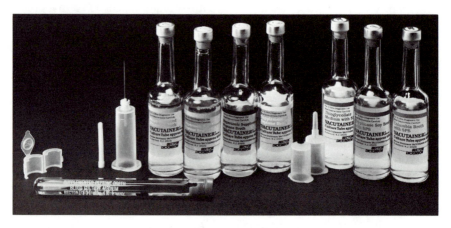

Figure 3–7. *(Courtesy of Becton-Dickinson and Co., Rutherford, NJ)*

120. If the phlebotomist collects only venipuncture specimens, which of the following items would not be needed on his or her specimen collection tray?

(A) alcohol, iodine, or Betadine pads
(B) disposable gloves
(C) lancets
(D) tourniquet

121. Which of the following anticoagulants is found in a green-stoppered blood collection vacuum tube?

    (A) EDTA
    (B) sodium heparin
    (C) sodium citrate
    (D) ammonium oxalate

122. Which of the following anticoagulants is found in a black-stoppered blood collection vacuum tube?

    (A) EDTA
    (B) sodium heparin
    (C) lithium heparin
    (D) sodium oxalate

123. Which of the following anticoagulants is found in a purple-stoppered blood collection vacuum tube?

    (A) EDTA
    (B) sodium heparin
    (C) ammonium oxalate
    (D) sodium oxalate

124. Which of the following anticoagulants is found in a royal blue-stoppered blood collection vacuum tube?

    (A) EDTA
    (B) sodium heparin
    (C) sodium citrate
    (D) ammonium heparin

DIRECTIONS: For each of the questions or incomplete statements below, ONE or MORE of the numbered responses are correct. In each case select:

    A. if only 1, 2, and 3 are correct
    B. if only 1 and 3 are correct
    C. if only 2 and 4 are correct
    D. if only 4 is correct
    E. if all are correct

125. A suitable lancet's puncturing tip for use on newborns must possess the appropriate

    (1) length
    (2) width
    (3) thickness
    (4) diameter

126. Which of the following must be included on the label of the blood specimen or body fluid specimen?

    ✓ (1) patient's name
    (2) patient's admission number
    (3) time specimen is collected
    (4) attending physician

127. To obtain a clean-catch urine specimen, the phlebotomist might need to explain which of the following to a female patient?

    ✓ (1) the woman should squeeze the skin folds together around the urinary opening
    (2) the skin folds around the urinary opening should be cleaned with a mild antiseptic soap and water
    (3) after collection, the urine specimen should be placed in a freezer until the analysis is performed
    (4) if the specimen is collected before the visit to the physician's office, the patient should label the container with her name and time of collection

DIRECTIONS: Each group of lettered words or phrases below is followed by a list of numbered words or phrases. MATCH the lettered word or phrase most closely associated with the numbered word or phrase.

Questions 128 through 132

A. general chemistry micro-collection
B. blood gases
C. RBC fragility test
D. lipid special stain
E. plasma (gray-stoppered blood collection tube)

128. B-D Unopette
129. Sulfa level
130. Needs mixing of microblood sample by use of a magnet
131. B-D Microtainer, polypropylene, 600 μL, silicon separator
132. Blood smear

Answers and Explanations

1. **C.** Sodium citrate anticoagulant is found in a blue-stoppered blood collecting vacuum tube.

    Garza D, Becan-McBride K. Phlebotomy Handbook. E. Norwalk, CT: Appleton & Lange; 1989:52.

2. **B.** Heparin is used to collect blood gases.

    Garza and Becan-McBride, p. 69.

3. **A.** The High Risk (HR) needle has been introduced to help the prevention of accidental needlesticks and transmission of AIDS.
   Garza and Becan-McBride, p 62.

4. **B.** If a blood specimen is allowed to clot, the result is serum plus blood cells meshed in a fibrin clot.
   Garza and Becan-McBride, p 44.

5. **B.** Cerebrospinal fluid (CSF) is obtained through a spinal tap or lumbar puncture.
   Garza and Becan-McBride, p 44.

6. **C.** Pancreatitis can be caused by corticosteroids, estrogens, and diuretics and causes an elevation of serum amylase.
   Garza and Becan-McBride, p 49.

7. **D.** Drug-induced hepatotoxicity (toxicity of the liver) can lead to an increase in the blood liver enzyme, alanine aminotransferase.
   Garza and Becan-McBride, p 49.

8. **E.** Some medications lead to renal (kidney) impairment, which will cause an elevation of blood urea nitrogen.
   Garza and Becan-McBride, p 49.

9. **B.** CAP is the abbreviated form of College of American Pathologists.
   Garza and Becan-McBride, p 49.

10. **A.** Drug interference leading to falsely decreased results in blood specimens may be caused by inhibition of the chromogenic or fluorescent reaction.
    Garza and Becan-McBride, p 47.

11. **B.** The anticoagulant EDTA is contained in the lavender-stoppered vacuum blood collection tube.
    Garza and Becan-McBride, p 51.

12. **D.** Potassium oxalate and sodium fluoride are contained in the gray-stoppered vacuum blood collection tube.
    Garza and Becan-McBride, p 51.

13. **A.** The additive lithium heparin is contained in the green-stoppered vacuum blood collection tube.
    Garza and Becan-McBride, p 51.

14. **E.** The royal blue-stoppered vacuum blood collection tube contains sodium heparin.
    Garza and Becan-McBride, p 51.

15. **C.** The gray and red-stoppered vacuum blood collection tube contains an inert polymer barrier.
    Garza and Becan-McBride, p 51.

16. **FALSE.** Sterile blood specimens are needed for blood cultures.
    Garza and Becan-McBride, p 53.

17. **TRUE.** The Datar resheather and tubeholder system decreases the possibility of accidental needlesticks and, thus, transmission of AIDS and other infectious diseases to phlebotomists.
    Garza and Becan-McBride, p 62.

18. **FALSE.** The gauge number indicates the diameter of the needle, but the smaller the number, the larger the needle.
    Garza and Becan-McBride, p 62.

19. **TRUE** Ethylenediaminetetraacetate usually is abbreviated as EDTA.
    Garza and Becan-McBride, p 52.

20. **FALSE.** The B-D Safety Lok needle holder is a device designed to encourage safer venipuncture technique. Following venipuncture, the protective shield slides and snaps into place, providing immediate containment of the used needle.
    Becton Dickinson Vacutainer Systems, Rutherford, NJ.

21. **FALSE.** Midstream urine specimens commonly are used for routine admission urinalysis.
    Garza and Becan-McBride, p 45.

22. **TRUE.** Pleural fluid is obtained from the lung cavity.
    Garza and Becan-McBride, p 44.

23. **FALSE.** Body fluids, such as pleural fluid, may be biohazardous, and the phlebotomist must be careful in the transportation of body fluids because they are difficult to obtain and may be biohazardous.
    Garza and Becan-McBride, p 44.

24. **TRUE.** Drug interference leading to falsely decreased results in blood specimens may be caused by the drug competing with the chromogenic reagent for peroxide in a peroxide-generating reaction, thus falsely decreasing the chromogen oxidation and concentration of the blood analyte.
    Garza and Becan-McBride, p 47.

25. **E.** Heparinized Natelson tubes (75 μL), disposable gloves, lancets, and alcohol or Betadine pads all are typically carried on a microcollection tray.
    Garza and Becan-McBride, p 73.

26. **E.** Blood collected through skin puncture is necessary for some adults who are severly burned, have veins that are difficult to stick because of their small size or location, are extremely obese, or have thrombotic tendencies.

    Becan-McBride, K. Specimen collection. In: Turgeon M, Terzian J, eds. Laboratory Medicine: Theory, Procedures and Applications. Boston: Little, Brown and Co; (In press).

27. **A.** Capillary blood collection systems include the Microvette capillary blood collection system (Sarstedt Inc., Princeton, NJ); the B-D Unopette (Becton-Dickinson and Co., Rutherford, NJ), and the B-D Microtainer (Becton-Dickinson and Co.).

    Garza and Becan-McBride, pp 70–72.

28. **E.** Tourniquets that are used in venipuncture include Penrose, strap, rubber hose, and blood pressure cuff.

    Garza and Becan-McBride, p 64.

29. **C.** Sodium citrate and sodium oxalate are used frequently in coagulation blood studies.

    Garza and Becan-McBride, pp 52–53.

30. **D.** Sodium heparin is used for clinical cytogenetic studies.

    Garza and Becan-McBride, p 52.

31. **E.** Gastric secretions, peritoneal fluid, pleural fluid, and cerebrospinal fluid (CSF) are fluids that the phlebotomist may be involved in transporting to the laboratory.

    Garza and Becan-McBride, p 44.

32. **C.** Chromosome analysis requires whole blood collected in a green-stoppered blood collection tube.

    Garza and Becan-McBride, p 55.

33. **A.** A blood cell count including WBC, RBC, hemoglobin (Hgb), hematocrit (Hct), mean corpuscular volume (MCV), mean corpuscular hemoglobin (MCH), and mean corpuscular hemoglobin concentration (MCHC) requires whole blood collected in a purple-stoppered blood collection tube.

    Garza and Becan-McBride, p 55.

34. **B.** The assay for the enzyme alkaline phosphatase usually requires serum collected in a red-stoppered blood collection tube.

    Garza and Becan-McBride, p 54.

35. **E.** The fasting blood glucose (FBG) test frequently requires plasma collected in a gray-stoppered blood collection tube.

    Garza and Becan-McBride, p 57.

36. **D.** Antithrombin III, a coagulation test, requires plasma collected in a blue-stoppered blood collection tube.
     Garza and Becan-McBride, p 54.

37. **C.** The butterfly is the most commonly used intravenous device that is sometimes used in the collection of blood from patients who are difficult to stick by conventional methods.
     Garza and Becan-McBride, p 64.

38. **B.** Heparinized Natelson tubes (75 μL) are used frequently for the microcollection of blood gases.
     Garza and Becan-McBride, p 70.

39. **D.** The Corvac tube (Monoject Scientific, a Division of Sherwood Medical) is a serum separation tube.
     Garza and Becan-McBride, pp 63, 65.

40. **E.** The B-D Microtainer tube (Becton-Dickinson and Co., Rutherford, NJ) is used frequently in the microcollection of electrolytes and general chemistry blood specimens.
     Garza and Becan-McBride, pp 69–70.

41. **A.** The B-D Unopette (Becton-Dickinson and Co., Rutherford, NJ) is a blood collection device prefilled with specific amounts of diluents or reagents.
     Garza and Becan-McBride, p 72.

42. **B.** Tylenol, or acetaminophen, can lead to falsely increased values in liver function tests.
     Garza and Becan-McBride, p 49.

43. **C.** Falsely decreased values of the blood analyte can be mistakenly interpreted as normal or subnormal if the blood analyte is truly in an elevated range or normal range, respectively.
     Garza and Becan-McBride, p 47.

44. **B.** The B-D Vacutainer System (Becton-Dickinson and Co., Rutherford, NJ) incorporates a blood collection vacuum tube to collect blood by venipuncture.
     Garza and Becan-McBride, pp 50–51.

45. **C.** Datar Inc. produces a no-cut needle disposal system (Figure 3–3) to discard needles and syringes and thus reduce the possibilities of needlesticks for the phlebotomists.
     Garza and Becan-McBride, pp 62–63.

46. **A.** Surgicutt (International Technidyne Corp., Edison, NJ) is a device to create uniform skin incisions for bleeding time.
     Garza and Becan-McBride, p 67.

47. **D.** Avoiding the use of gloves with talc powder when collecting blood is recommended because the tubes of patients' blood may become contaminated with this powder, leading to falsely elevated calcium values.

    Garza and Becan-McBride, p 67.

48. **D.** Blood for assay of the enzyme alkaline phosphatase usually is collected in a red-stoppered blood collection vacuum tube.

    Garza and Becan-McBride, p 54.

49. **B.** The blood for the hematocrit test usually is collected in a purple-stoppered blood collection vacuum tube.

    Garza and Becan-McBride, p 57.

50. **A.** The sedimentation rate (ESR) requires whole blood collected in a purple-stoppered blood collection vacuum tube.

    Garza and Becan-McBride, p 60.

51. **D.** The lead assay requires blood collected in a dark blue-stoppered blood collection vacuum tube.

    Garza and Becan-McBride, p 58.

52. **A.** In pediatric collections, disposable sterile lancets with tips of 2.4 mm or less in length, such as provided by the Monolet, are required to avoid penetrating bone.

    Meites S. Skin puncture and blood collecting techniques for infants: update and problems. Clin Chem. *1988;34:1890–1894.*

53. **B.** Falsely increased laboratory results for the blood analyte can be mistakenly interpreted as elevated or normal if the blood analyte is truly in a normal range or decreased range, respectively.

    Garza and Becan-McBride, pp 48–49.

54. **FALSE.** This is a photograph of a blood microcollection vial manufactured by Sherwood Medical, St. Louis, Mo. B-D Unopette (Becton-Dickinson and Co., Rutherford, NJ) is a collection and dilution device.

    Garza and Becan-McBride, pp 70–72.

55. **TRUE.** The Autolet is a spring-activated puncture device with two disposable platforms for control of penetration depth.

    Garza and Becan-McBride, pp 68–69.

56. **FALSE.** The phlebotomist is the link between the clinical laboratory and the patient. Thus, the phlebotomist should write a note on the laboratory requisition slip indicating that the patient stated during blood collection that he or she had taken numerous aspirin over the past 2 days.

    Garza and Becan-McBride, pp 49–50.

57. **TRUE.** Blood collection vacuum tubes usually contain silicon to decrease the possibility of hemolysis and prevent the clot from adhering to the wall of the tube.
    Garza and Becan-McBride, p 51.

58. **FALSE.** Aerotrap is used in laboratories to remove the stopper from vacuum tubes.
    Garza and Becan-McBride, p 53.

59. **TRUE.** Sterile vacuum collection tubes are used frequently for trace element studies.
    Garza and Becan-McBride, p 53.

60. **TRUE.** Citrate phosphate dextrose (CPD) is an anticoagulant used in the collection of blood for blood donations.
    Garza and Becan-McBride, p 52.

61. **FALSE.** Sputum is fluid from the lungs, containing pus.
    Garza and Becan-McBride, p 46.

62. **FALSE.** Serum is obtained from whole blood that is not mixed with any anticoagulant.
    Garza and Becan-McBride, p 43.

63. **TRUE.** Heparin is a mucopolysaccharide used in assays, for example, for ammonia and plasma hemoglobin.
    Garza and Becan-McBride, p 52.

64. **C.** The Hemalet has an automatic blade retraction mechanism used to create skin incisions for bleeding time.
    Garza and Becan-McBride, p 67.

65. **B.** The total estrogens assay is run on serum collected in a red-stopped vacuum tube.
    Garza and Becan-McBride, p 56.

66. **A.** The erythrocyte fragility test requires whole blood collected in a purple-stoppered vacuum tube.
    Garza and Becan-McBride, p 56.

67. **E.** The leukocyte alkaline phosphatase stain requires six fresh blood smears.
    Garza and Becan-McBride, p 58.

68. **D.** The renin activity assay requires whole blood collected in a purple-stoppered vacuum tube and transported on ice.
    Garza and Becan-McBride, p 60.

69. **D.** The enzyme aspartate aminotransferase (AST) is the same as SGOT.
    Garza and Becan-McBride, p 60.

70. **E.** The sucrose presumptive test is abbreviated PNH (paroxysmal nocturnal hemoglobinuria).
    Garza and Becan-McBride, p 60.

71. **A.** The enzyme alanine aminotransferase (ALT) is the same as SGPT.
    Garza and Becan-McBride, p 60.

72. **C.** APTT is the abbreviation for activated thromboplastin time.
    Garza and Becan-McBride, p 61.

73. **B.** ESR is the abbreviated term for sedimentation rate.
    Garza and Becan-McBride, p 56.

74. **A.** FBS, fasting blood glucose, and glucose are the same assay, and, thus, all are collected in a gray-stoppered vacuum tube.
    Garza and Becan-McBride, p 57.

75. **E.** Sterile vacuum collecting tubes are used frequently in the following determinations: prothrombin (PT), sedimentation rate (ESR), trace element studies, and activated clotting time.
    Garza and Becan-McBride, p 53.

76. **D.** Bilirubin is light sensitive and will decrease in value if the blood for its collection is exposed to light.
    Garza and Becan-McBride, p 75.

77. **D.** Fibrinogen is found in plasma but is removed from serum during the clotting process.
    Garza and Becan-McBride, p 43.

78. **B.** For the platelet function profile, whole blood collected in a purple-stoppered vacuum tube and whole blood in a blue-stoppered vacuum tube are needed.
    Garza and Becan-McBride, p 59.

79. **A.** Russell viper venom time, also expressed as RVV or Stypven time, is run on plasma collected in a blue-stoppered blood collection tube.
    Garza and Becan-McBride, p 60.

80. **B.** Blood tests to detect syphilis are the RPR test and the VDRL test.
    Garza, and Becan-McBride, pp. 60–61.

81. **A.** Thyroid-stimulating hormone (TSH) and thyroxine (T_4) are procedures specifically to test for thyroid functioning.
    Garza and Becan-McBride, pp 60–61.

82. **D.** Needles for vacuum tubes and syringes are not needed on a tray to collect microcollection specimens.
    Garza and Becan-McBride, p 73.

83. **TRUE.** Figure 3–6 is the B-D Unopette, a collection and dilution unit for blood samples.
    Garza and Becan-McBride, p 72.

84. **FALSE.** Patients should not be allowed to submit urine specimens in their own jars because they may not be chemically clean and do not contain the required preservatives.
    Garza and Becan-McBride, p 45.

85. **FALSE.** The first step in the collection process of a 24-hour urine specimen should begin between 6 and 8 AM, with the exact time written on the container label.
    Garza and Becan-McBride, p 46.

86. **TRUE.** Pericardial fluid is obtained from the heart cavity.
    Garza and Becan-McBride, p 44.

87. **TRUE.** The fluorescent treponemal antibody test is also referred to as MHA-TP.
    Garza and Becan-McBride, p 57.

88. **FALSE** The low-density lipoproteins assay sometimes is abbreviated on the test requisition as LDL.
    Garza and Becan-McBride, p 59.

89. **TRUE.** The Valium test sometimes is referred to as the diazepam assay.
    Garza and Becan-McBride, p 61.

90. **FALSE.** HAA is an abbreviation for hepatitis-associated antigen.
    Garza and Becan-McBride, p 61.

91. **TRUE.** PAS for glycogen is a special stain procedure and requires a blood smear.
    Garza and Becan-McBride, p 60.

92. **TRUE.** The laboratory test Monospot is the same as the heterophil antibody test and requires serum collected in a red-stoppered blood collection tube.
    Garza and Becan-McBride, p 58.

93. **TRUE.** If the phlebotomist had to collect blood for the Dilantin assay, the blood specimen could be used for the phenytoin assay, since Dilantin and phenytoin are the same.
    Garza and Becan-McBride, p 59.

94. **E.** The vitamin D (25-OH) assay requires whole blood collected in a purple-stoppered blood collection tube.
Garza and Becan-McBride, p 61.

95. **B.** BUN is the same as blood urea nitrogen or urea nitrogen.
Garza and Becan-McBride, p 61.

96. **A.** The thiamine assay requires whole blood collected in a green-stoppered blood collection tube.
Garza and Becan-McBride, p 60.

97. **C.** Thrombin time requires plasma collected in a blue-stoppered blood collection tube.
Garza and Becan-McBride, p 60.

98. **D.** The sucrose presumptive test requires whole blood collected in a blue-stoppered blood collection tube.
Garza and Becan-McBride, p 60.

99. **C.** The glycolytic action of the blood cells interferes in the analysis of glucose. Thus, the blood samples must be transported to the clinical laboratory as soon as possible.
Garza and Becan-McBride, pp 74–75.

100. **D.** Microbiology blood specimens must be transported to culture media as quickly as possible.
Garza and Becan-McBride, p 75.

101. **A.** For the insulin test, the tube of blood must be placed in an ice container immediately after collection.
Garza and Becan-McBride, p 58.

102. **E.** The Heinz bodies special stain requires a blood smear.
Garza and Becan-McBride, p 60.

103. **B.** For the bilirubin assay, the blood must be protected from light.
Garza and Becan-McBride, p 75.

104. **C.** The E-rosette test requires whole blood collected in a purple-stoppered blood collection tube.
Garza and Becan-McBride, p 56.

105. **D.** Renin activity requires plasma collected in a purple-stoppered blood collection tube.
Garza and Becan-McBride, p 60.

106. **E.** Ferritin requires serum collected in a red-stoppered blood collection tube.
Garza and Becan-McBride, p 57.

107.   **A.** The Coombs test requires a whole blood sample collected in a red-stoppered blood collection tube.
Garza and Becan-McBride, p 56.

108.   **B.** Factor assays require plasma collected in a blue-stoppered blood collection tube.
Garza and Becan-McBride, p 57.

109.   **A.** The B-D Unopette (Becton-Dickinson and Co., Rutherford, NJ) has a plastic reservoir containing a premeasured volume of reagent for diluting, has a reusable, self-filling diluting pipette, and consists of a straight, thin-wall uniform-bore glass capillary tube fitted into a plastic holder.
Garza and Becan-McBride, p 72.

110.   **E.** Zinc, transaminase, testosterone, and rubella are all collected in a red-stoppered blood collection tube to obtain serum.
Garza and Becan-McBride, pp 60–61.

111.   **A.** Gray-stoppered blood collection tubes can be ordered containing potassium oxalate and sodium fluoride, sodium fluoride and thymol, or potassium oxalate.
Garza and Becan-McBride, p 52.

112.   **B.** The blood cell count, including the differential and Heinz bodies special stain, requires a blood smear.
Garza and Becan-McBride, pp 55, 60.

113.   **C.** The A/G ratio refers to the albumin/globulin ratio.
Garza and Becan-McBride, p 61.

114.   **D.** The serum must be separated from the red blood cells and white blood cells as quickly as possible to avoid glycolysis, which will falsely decrease the glucose value.
Garza and Becan-McBride, p 52.

115.   **E.** For determination of ammonia, chromosome analysis, cryofibrinogen, and the LE cell test, blood must be collected in a green-stoppered blood collection tube.
Garza and Becan-McBride, pp 54–58.

116.   **A.** The volume of plasma or serum that generally can be collected from a premature infant is approximately 100 to 150 μL, and about two times that amount from a full-term newborn. Larger volumes are obtained from older children and adults.
Garza and Becan-McBride, p 68.

117.   **A.** Maximum length of 5 mm is the best for older children.
Garza and Becan-McBride, p 68.

118. **C.** When blood clots, the centrifuged blood has serum that contains no fibrinogen. However, the blood cells are at the bottom of the tube in the fibrin clot.
Garza and Becan-McBride, p 44.

119. **D.** The tubes in Figure 3–7 are B-D Vacutainer Microbiology Specimen Collection Units.
Garza and Becan-McBride, p 53.

120. **C.** Lancets for skin puncture would not be needed on the specimen collection tray belonging to the phlebotomist who only collects venipuncture specimens.
Garza and Becan-McBride, p 73.

121. **B.** The anticoagulant sodium heparin is found in a green-stoppered blood collection vacuum tube.
Garza and Becan-McBride, p 52.

122. **D.** The anticoagulant sodium oxalate is found in a black-stoppered blood collection vacuum tube.
Garza and Becan-McBride, p 53.

123. **A.** The anticoagulant EDTA is found in a purple-stoppered blood collection vacuum tube.
Garza and Becan-McBride, p 52.

124. **B.** The anticoagulant sodium heparin is found in a royal blue-stoppered blood collection tube.
Garza and Becan-McBride, p 52.

125. **E.** A suitable lancet's puncturing tip for use on newborns must possess appropriate length, appropriate width and thickness, and appropriate diameter.
Meites, pp 1890–1894.

126. **E.** The label on the blood specimen or body fluid specimen must include the patient's name, patient's admission number, time specimen is collected, attending physician, date, and type of specimen.
Garza and Becan-McBride, p 44.

127. **C.** The woman should separate the skin folds around the urinary opening. Holding the skin folds apart, she should clean the area with a mild antiseptic soap and water. Next, holding the skin folds apart with one hand and after urinating into the toilet, the patient should urinate into a sterile container. The patient must label the container with her name and time of collection. The specimen must be refrigerated immediately if the analysis is not performed right after the collection.
Garza and Becan-McBride, p 45.

128. **C.** The B-D Unopette is used for the RBC fragility test.
    Garza and Becan-McBride, p 72.

129. **E.** The sulfa level sample must be collected in a gray-stoppered blood collection tube to obtain plasma.
    Garza and Becan-McBride, p 60.

130. **B.** The microcollection of blood gases requires mixing the sample by use of a magnet.
    Garza and Becan-McBride, p 70.

131. **A.** The B-D Microtainer is used frequently for the collection of general chemistry microspecimens.
    Garza and Becan-McBride, p 69.

132. **D.** The lipid special stain requires a blood smear.
    Garza and Becan-McBride, p 60.

CHAPTER 4

Collection Procedures and Physiologic Complications

Questions

DIRECTIONS: Indicate whether each statement is TRUE or FALSE.

1. **True/False:** Basal state requires an overnight fast (12 to 14 hours).
2. **True/False:** Blood composition is significantly altered after meals.
3. **True/False:** Some laboratory tests are affected by excessive exercise.
4. **True/False:** Basal state means the body is in a reclining position.
5. **True/False:** If a specimen collection procedure involves some discomfort, the patient must not be informed.
6. **True/False:** Lipemic serum is serum in the basal state.
7. **True/False:** Coffee and tea should be avoided when fasting.
8. **True/False:** Turbid or cloudy serum can be due to bacterial contamination.
9. **True/False:** Age and pregnancy have an effect on laboratory values.
10. **True/False:** Laboratory reference ranges are often cited according to age.
11. **True/False:** Most patients are very relaxed when they are to have their blood collected.
12. **True/False:** Exercise can cause some enzymes to remain elevated in the blood for up to 24 hours.
13. **True/False:** Anxiety can cause elevations in white cell counts.
14. **True/False:** Gender can affect laboratory results.
15. **True/False:** Hair color can affect some laboratory results.
16. **True/False:** Some chemical constituents are changed in the blood when a patient moves from a lying position to a standing position.
17. **True/False:** Hyperventilation can cause changes in laboratory tests.
18. **True/False:** Hospitalized patients should wear an identification bracelet.
19. **True/False:** Misidentification of a patient's specimen can result in death of another patient.

20. **True/False:** An employee who misidentifies a specimen may be dismissed from employment.

21. **True/False:** Specimen containers should be prelabeled before blood collection.

22. **True/False:** Butterfly needles are used only for collecting arterial blood gases.

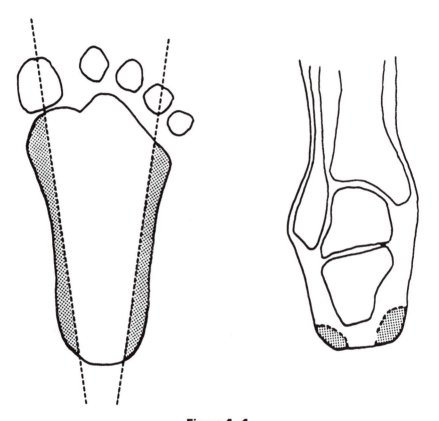

Figure 4–1.

23. **True/False:** The shaded areas in Figure 4–1 indicate the most hazardous sites for performing heel punctures on children.

24. **True/False:** The first drop of blood after a fingerstick is the most valuable for assessing laboratory values.

25. **True/False:** A decontaminated site for venipuncture should not be touched with a nonsterile object.

26. **True/False:** Patients should be reassured that a venipuncture will not hurt.

27. **True/False:** During venipuncture, the needle should be inserted with the bevel side downward.
28. **True/False:** During a venipuncture, the tourniquet should be released before the needle is withdrawn.
29. **True/False:** A fingerstick puncture should be across the fingerprint not parallel to the fingerprint.

DIRECTIONS: Each group of lettered words or phrases below is followed by a list of numbered words or phrases. MATCH the lettered word or phrase most closely associated with the numbered word or phrase.

Questions 30 through 34

A. LDH   30. Creatinine phosphokinase
B. CDC   31. Erythrocyte
C. RBC   32. Lactate dehydrogenase
D. CPK   33. Centers for Disease Control
E. AST   34. Aspartate amino transferase

Questions 35 through 39

A. supine   35. Eating food
B. lipemic   36. Cloudy
C. diurnal rhythms   37. Lying position
D. fasting   38. Body fluid fluctuations during the day
E. nonfasting   39. Abstaining from food

Questions 40 through 43

A. 70% isopropanol   40. Used for decontamination before blood collec-
B. ether   tion for hematology tests
C. povidone-iodine   41. Used for decontamination before blood collec-
D. cholesterol   tion for blood cultures
                     42. Blood test usually performed in a chemistry
                            laboratory
                     43. A hazardous laboratory chemical

Questions 44 through 47

A. occluded veins   44. Small red spots in the skin
B. syncope   45. Fainting

C. petechiae   46. Blood leaking into tissues
D. hematoma   47. Blocked veins

DIRECTIONS: Indicate whether each statement is TRUE or FALSE.

48. True/False: Alcohol present on a finger during a fingerstick can prevent a round drop of blood from forming.

49. True/False: Capillary pipettes fill by capillary action.

50. True/False: When making blood smears on a glass slide, it is best to
use freshly collected blood.

51. True/False: To speed the drying of a blood smear, a phlebotomist
should blow on the slide.

52. True/False: When filling a capillary tube with blood, it is important
not to have air bubbles.

53. True/False: A phlebotomist is responsible for checking the puncture
site afterward to assure that the bleeding has stopped.

54. True/False: Most patients are allergic to iodine.

**DIRECTIONS: For each of the questions or incomplete statements below,
ONE or MORE of the numbered responses are correct. In each case select**

A. if only 1, 2, and 3 are correct
B. if only 1 and 3 are correct
C. if only 2 and 4 are correct
D. if only 4 is correct
E. if all are correct

55. Which of the following will cause changes in a basal state?

(1) tourniquet application
(2) stress and drugs
(3) exercise
(4) diet

56. If a patient has eaten just before collection of a blood sample, what
should the phlebotomist do?

(1) collect the specimen
(2) indicate what the patient ate
(3) make a note that the patient was "nonfasting"
(4) avoid collecting the specimen

57. The term "fasting" usually means

(1) abstaining from water
(2) abstaining from everything

(3) abstaining from smoking
(4) abstaining from food and drinks other than water

58. The word "nonfasting" should be indicated on the specimen or requisition form under which of the listed circumstances?

(1) if the patient did not have breakfast
(2) if the patient ate breakfast
(3) if the patient needs a blood glucose level
(4) if the patient ate a small snack

59. The term "fasting" refers to abstaining from

(1) food
(2) coffee
(3) chewing gum
(4) water

60. Normally, serum is described as

(1) clear
(2) milky
(3) light yellow or straw-colored
(4) red

61. What is the best way to identify a patient before venipuncture?

(1) ask the patient his or her name
(2) state the name, then ask the patient if it is correct
(3) check the identification bracelet
(4) review the medical chart

62. If a patient does not have an identification bracelet, what should be done?

(1) a doctor should cancel the tests
(2) a nurse in charge of the patient should make the identification
(3) the phlebotomist should go ahead and draw the blood
(4) documentation of the nurse who made the identification should be noted

63. Ambulatory patient identity should be confirmed by

(1) checking a drivers license
(2) asking that a relative and nurse document the identity
(3) verifying the birth date
(4) checking the fingerprint

64. A labeled specimen must include

    (1) name and ID number
    (2) time of collection
    (3) phlebotomist's initials
    (4) date of collection

65. A laboratory requisition must include

    (1) date and time of request
    (2) hospital room number or bed assignment
    (3) patient's name and ID number
    (4) patient's physician

66. Before a venipuncture, a phlebotomist should

    (1) prepare himself or herself emotionally
    (2) prepare all supplies and equipment needed
    (3) put on clean gloves
    (4) talk to the patient's physician

67. A phlebotomist should not use arm veins in which of the following circumstances?

    (1) if the patient has an IV in both arms
    (2) if the patient has a cast
    (3) if the patient has edematous arms
    (4) if burns are present on the arms

68. Which of the following veins are used most frequently for venipunctures?

    (1) cephalic vein
    (2) basilic vein
    (3) median cubital vein
    (4) aorta

69. Lipemic sera can be due to

    (1) ingestion of alcohol
    (2) bacterial contamination
    (3) excessive fasting
    (4) ingestion of fatty substances

70. For timed blood glucose levels, the patient must

    (1) abstain from food for 2 hours
    (2) abstain from water for 5 hours

(3) take deep breaths before the venipuncture

(4) abstain from food for 12–14 hours

71. Which of the following can affect laboratory tests on blood specimens?

 (1) altitude
 (2) temperature
 (3) humidity
 (4) geographic location

72. Which of the listed items can affect laboratory results?

 (1) sneezing
 (2) violent crying
 (3) smiling
 (4) medications

73. Good skin puncture site(s) include

 (1) the middle toe
 (2) the middle finger
 (3) the wrist
 (4) medial or lateral sections of the bottom surface of the heel

74. Complications resulting from multiple deep skin punctures on an infant's heel include

 (1) hepatitis
 (2) AIDS
 (3) pneumonia
 (4) osteomyelitis

75. Which of the following conditions has an adverse effect on the quality of a fingerstick?

 (1) swollen fingers
 (2) excessive milking of the finger
 (3) using the first drop of blood
 (4) the presence of a wedding ring

76. A tourniquet applied to the arm before a venipuncture must be done under what circumstances?

 (1) it should be comfortable to the patient
 (2) it should be tied for easy release
 (3) it should not be left more than 60 seconds
 (4) it should be clean

77. Phlebotomists can cause hemolysis by which of the following actions?

(1) slowly inverting the specimen tubes for mixing
(2) forcing blood into a test tube from a syringe
(3) using a butterfly needle for a venipuncture
(4) vigorously shaking the specimen tubes

78. Which of the following circumstances result in failure to draw blood during a venipuncture?

(1) needle is inserted through the vein
(2) losing the vacuum in the specimen tube
(3) veins are sclerosed
(4) tourniquet is too tight

79. Which of the following would be reason to reject a specimen for testing?

(1) use of expired collection tubes
(2) unlabeled specimen tubes
(3) discrepancies on a requisition
(4) incorrect collection tube used

80. Which of the following is NOT a suitable site for skin puncture?

(1) finger
(2) ankle and wrist
(3) heel
(4) earlobe

81. An ideal fingerstick should include which of the following steps?

(1) decontamination
(2) puncture in one sharp continuous motion
(3) perpendicular to the site and across the fingerprint
(4) wiping of the first drop

82. Blood smears for evaluation of cells should have which of the following characteristics?

(1) approximately one half of the slide should be covered
(2) it should have a feathered edge
(3) there should be no ridges, lines, or holes
(4) there should be no residual blood on the slide

83. Complications of a phlebotomy procedure include which of the following?

    (1) hematomas
    (2) alterations in the basal state
    (3) syncope
    (4) headaches

84. Hemoconcentration can be caused by

    (1) tourniquet application for extended periods
    (2) squeezing or probing a site
    (3) long-term IV therapy
    (4) sclerosed or occluded veins

DIRECTIONS: Each of the questions or incomplete statements below is followed by suggested answers or completions. Select the BEST answer in each case.

85. Basal state is best described as

    (A) after evening meal
    (B) before lunch
    (C) 3 hours after lunch
    (D) early morning, 12 hours after last food ingestion

86. Laboratory results are nonreliable if

    (A) normal values are not calculated
    (B) specimens are collected during basal state
    (C) specimens are collected after dinner
    (D) specimens are collected after ingestion of water

87. Normally, serum is what color?

    (A) pink and cloudy
    (B) red and thick
    (C) clear, light yellow, or straw-colored
    (D) clear, brownish red

88. What is the best position for the patient to be in during a venipuncture procedure?

    (A) standing over a counter
    (B) sitting on a work stool
    (C) reclining on a bed
    (D) sitting on the edge of a bed

89. A skin puncture on an infant's heel should not be more than how deep?

    (A) 1 cm
    (B) 2.4 mm
    (C) 2.4 cm
    (D) 1.5 mm

90. Which of the listed sequences is the BEST method for performing a fingerstick?

    (A) squeeze the finger, decontaminate, puncture the skin
    (B) decontaminate, squeeze the finger, puncture the skin, collect the first drop
    (C) decontaminate, puncture the skin, wipe first drop, collect blood sample
    (D) apply tourniquet, puncture the skin, wipe first drop, collect blood sample

91. Warming a site for venipuncture or skin puncture has what effect?

    (A) increases blood pressure
    (B) increases blood flow to the site
    (C) relaxes the patient
    (D) eliminates the need for a tourniquet

92. The best angle for spreading a blood smear using two glass slides is

    (A) 90 degrees
    (B) 180 degrees
    (C) 50 degrees
    (D) 30 degrees

93. The best angle for needle insertion into a vein is

    (A) 15 degrees
    (B) 30 degrees
    (C) 45 degrees
    (D) 90 degrees

Answers

1. TRUE.

   Garza D, Becan-McBride K. Phlebotomy Handbook. E. Norwalk, CT: Appleton & Lange, 1989:80.

2. **TRUE.**
    Garza and Becan-McBride, p 80.

3. **TRUE.**
    Garza and Becan-McBride, p 81.

4. **FALSE.**
    Garza and Becan-McBride, p 80.

5. **FALSE.**
    Garza and Becan-McBride, p 95.

6. **FALSE.**
    Garza and Becan-McBride, p 80.

7. **TRUE.**
    Garza and Becan-McBride, p 80.

8. **TRUE.**
    Garza and Becan-McBride, p 80.

9. **TRUE.**
    Garza and Becan-McBride, p 81.

10. **TRUE.**
    Garza and Becan-McBride, p 81.

11. **FALSE.**
    Garza and Becan-McBride, p 81.

12. **TRUE.**
    Garza and Becan-McBride, p 81.

13. **TRUE.**
    Garza and Becan-McBride, p 81.

14. **TRUE.**
    Garza and Becan-McBride, p 81.

15. **FALSE.**
    Garza and Becan-McBride, p 81.

16. **TRUE.**
    Garza and Becan-McBride, p 81.

17. **TRUE.**
    Garza and Becan-McBride, p 81.

18. **TRUE.**
    Garza and Becan-McBride, p 82.

19. **TRUE.**
    Garza and Becan-McBride, p 82.

20. **TRUE.**
    Garza and Becan-McBride, p 82.

21. **FALSE.**
    Garza and Becan-McBride, p 84.

22. **FALSE.**
    Garza and Becan-McBride, p 91.

23. **FALSE.**
    Garza and Becan-McBride, p 88.

24. **FALSE.**
    Garza and Becan-McBride, p 90.

25. **TRUE.**
    Garza and Becan-McBride, p 91.

26. **FALSE.**
    Garza and Becan-McBride, p 95.

27. **FALSE.**
    Garza and Becan-McBride, p 94.

28. **TRUE.**
    Garza and Becan-McBride, p 94.

29. **TRUE.**
    Garza and Becan-McBride, p 98.

30. **D.**
    Garza and Becan-McBride, pp 297–308.

31. **C.**
    Garza and Becan-McBride, pp 297–308.

32. **A.**
    Garza and Becan-McBride, pp 297–308.

33. **B.**
    Garza and Becan-McBride, pp 297–308.

34. **E.**
    Garza and Becan-McBride, pp 297–308.

35. **E.**
    Garza and Becan-McBride, pp 80–81.

36. **B.**
    Garza and Becan-McBride, pp 80–81.

37. **A.**
    Garza and Becan-McBride, pp 80–81.

38. **C.**
    Garza and Becan-McBride, pp 80–81.

39. **D.**
    Garza and Becan-McBride, pp 80–81.

40. **A.**
    Garza and Becan-McBride, p 91.

41. **C.**
    Garza and Becan-McBride, p 91.

42. **D.**

43. **B.**

44. **C.**
    Garza and Becan-McBride, p 107.

45. **B.**
    Garza and Becan-McBride, p 107.

46. **D.**
    Garza and Becan-McBride, p 107.

47. **A.**
    Garza and Becan-McBride, p 107.

48. **TRUE.**
    Garza and Becan-McBride, p 101.

49. **TRUE.**
    Garza and Becan-McBride, p 101.

50. **TRUE.**
    Garza and Becan-McBride, p 100.

51. **FALSE.**
    Garza and Becan-McBride, p 101.

52. **TRUE.**
    Garza and Becan-McBride, p 102.

53. **TRUE.**
    Garza and Becan-McBride, p 102.

54. **FALSE.**

    Garza and Becan-McBride, p 107.

55. **E.**

    Garza and Becan-McBride, pp 80–81.

56. **B.**

    Garza and Becan-McBride, pp 80–81.

57. **D.**

    Garza and Becan-McBride, p 80.

58. **C.**

    Garza and Becan-McBride, p 80.

59. **A.**

    Garza and Becan-McBride, p 80.

60. **B.**

    Garza and Becan-McBride, p 80.

61. **B.**

    Garza and Becan-McBride, p 82.

62. **C.**

    Garza and Becan-McBride, p 82.

63. **A.**

    Garza and Becan-McBride, p 82.

64. **E.**

    Garza and Becan-McBride, pp 82–84.

65. **E.**

    Garza and Becan-McBride, pp 82–84.

66. **A.**

    Garza and Becan-McBride, pp 84–85.

67. **E.**

    Garza and Becan-McBride, p 85.

68. **A.**

    Garza and Becan-McBride, p 85.

69. **C.**

    Garza and Becan-McBride, p 80.

70. **D.**

    Garza and Becan-McBride, p 80.

71. **E.**
Garza and Becan-McBride, pp 80–82.

72. **C.**
Garza and Becan-McBride, p 80–82.

73. **C.**
Garza and Becan-McBride, p 88.

74. **D.**
Garza and Becan-McBride, p 88.

75. **A.**
Garza and Becan-McBride, pp 100–102.

76. **E.**
Garza and Becan-McBride, p 91.

77. **C.**
Garza and Becan-McBride, p 94.

78. **A.**
Garza and Becan-McBride, p 103.

79. **E.**
Garza and Becan-McBride, p 110.

80. **C.**
Garza and Becan-McBride, p 88.

81. **E.**
Garza and Becan-McBride, p 101.

82. **A.**
Garza and Becan-McBride, p 100.

83. **B.**
Garza and Becan-McBride, p 103.

84. **E.**
Garza and Becan-McBride, p 107.

85. **D.**
Garza and Becan-McBride, p 80.

86. **C.**
Garza and Becan-McBride, p 80.

87. **C.**
Garza and Becan-McBride, p 80.

88. **C.**

    Garza and Becan-McBride, p 85.

89. **B.**

    Garza and Becan-McBride, p 88.

90. **C.**

    Garza and Becan-McBride, p 98.

91. **B.**

    Garza and Becan-McBride, p 90.

92. **D.**

    Garza and Becan-McBride, p 100.

93. **A.**

    Garza and Becan-McBride, p 94.

CHAPTER 5

Special Collection Procedures

Questions

DIRECTIONS: Each of the questions or incomplete statements below is followed by suggested answers or completions. Select the BEST answer in each case.

1. Which of the following is the specimen of choice for testing the pH, Po_2, and Pco_2 of the blood?

   (A) skin puncture blood
   (B) venous blood
   (C) heparinized plasma
   (D) arterial blood

2. Which of the following sites is NOT recommended to collect capillary blood gases?

   (A) lateral posterior area of the heel
   (B) lateral anterior area of the elbow
   (C) the great toe
   (D) the ball of the finger

3. What should be the minimum volume of the capillary tube used to collect a specimen for capillary blood gas analysis?

   (A) 25 μL
   (B) 50 μL
   (C) 100 μL
   (D) 200 μL

4. Which of the following arteries in the leg is recommended for drawing blood for arterial blood gases?

   (A) brachial artery
   (B) femoral artery

(C) radial artery

(D) lateral posterior artery

5. Which of the following is required to collect blood for the arterial blood gases?

(A) Penrose tourniquet

(B) rubber hose tourniquet

(C) no tourniquet

(D) blood pressure cuff

6. The required amount of sample for arterial blood gases collected with a syringe and needle is about

(A) 1 mL

(B) 5 mL

(C) 7 mL

(D) 10 mL

7. Which of the following is a useful tool for testing platelet plug formation in the capillaries?

(A) bleeding time test

(B) arterial blood gases

(C) glucose tolerance test

(D) D-xylose test

8. The bleeding time test is performed by making a minor standardized incision in either the

(A) earlobe or hand

(B) forearm or radial artery in leg

(C) foot or forearm

(D) earlobe or forearm

DIRECTIONS: For each of the questions or incomplete statements below, ONE or MORE of the numbered responses are correct. In each case select

A. if only 1, 2, and 3 are correct
B. if only 1 and 3 are correct
C. if only 2 and 4 are correct
D. if only 4 is correct
E. if all are correct

9. A prolonged bleeding time for a patient may be caused by the patient's intake of

(1) aspirin

(2) mithramycin

(3) ethyl alcohol
(4) dextran

10. Instead of running the Lee-White clotting time test, which of the following assays is/are better assays for coagulation factor deficiencies?

(1) prothrombin time
(2) PT
(3) activated partial thromboplastin time
(4) PTT

11. Which of the following items is/are needed to collect a blood culture specimen?

(1) disposable gloves
(2) iodine scrub swabstick
(3) alcohol preps
(4) four B-D Unopettes

12. For the epinephrine tolerance test, blood is collected to test for

(1) blood urea nitrogen
(2) blood sugar
(3) epinephrine
(4) glucose

13. The sweat chloride test is used in the diagnosis of

(1) muscular dystrophy
(2) diabetes mellitus
(3) diabetes insipidus
(4) cystic fibrosis

14. Which of the following dye(s) has/have been used to test a patient's liver function?

(1) cardiogreen dye
(2) indocyanine green dye
(3) Bromsulphalein dye
(4) phenosulphalein dye

15. Blood glucose levels are measured on patients having which of the following assays performed?

(1) glucagon tolerance test
(2) epinephrine tolerance test
(3) lactose tolerance test
(4) D-xylose tolerance test

DIRECTIONS: Each group of lettered words or phrases below is followed by a list of numbered words or phrases. MATCH the lettered word or phrase most closely associated with the numbered word or phrase.

Questions 16 through 20

A. skin test
B. epinephrine tolerance test
C. D-xylose tolerance test
D. pilocarpine hydrochloric acid (HCl)
E. nasopharyngeal culture

16. Cystic fibrosis
17. Whooping cough
18. Tuberculin syringe
19. von Gierke's disease
20. Malabsorption disease

Questions 21 through 25

A. Hollander test
B. Surgicutt
C. Blood culture
D. GTT
E. Therapeutic drug monitoring

21. Fevers of unknown origin
22. Diabetes mellitus
23. Trough and peak levels
24. Determines gastric function in terms of stomach acid production
25. Bleeding time

DIRECTIONS: Indicate whether each statement is TRUE or FALSE.

26. **True/False:** A second site blood culture is a very effective tool for routine blood culture orders and provides a great amount of information that properly spaced, timed blood cultures cannot provide.
27. **True/False:** Most blood cultures require 3 to 5 mL of blood per bottle.
28. **True/False:** The 2-hour postprandial glucose test can be used to screen patients for diabetes.
29. **True/False:** In order to donate blood, a donor must weigh at least 125 pounds.
30. **True/False:** The term STAT means immediately.
31. **True/False:** It is recommended that blood for serum iron be drawn after other specimens are collected in tubes with EDTA.
32. **True/False:** The capillary tube and items in Figure 5–1 are used to collect arterial blood gases.

CAPILLARY TUBE

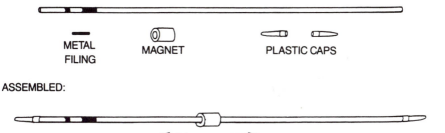

Figure 5—1. *From Garza, D., and Becan McBride, K.* Phlebotomy Handbook, second edition. *Appleton & Lange: Norwalk, Ct; 1989.*

33. **True/False:** In the Surgicutt bleeding time test, the phlebotomist must wick the flow of blood with filter paper every 30 seconds until blood no longer stains the paper.

34. **True/False:** For blood donations, the hematocrit must be no less than 30% for female donors.

35. **True/False:** The most common requests for timed blood specimens are hemoglobin levels drawn 2 hours after a meal.

36. **True/False:** Any blood vacuum collection tube that has an anticoagulant in it should be drawn first when multiple blood assays are requested on a patient.

DIRECTIONS: Each of the questions or incomplete statements below is followed by suggested answers or completions. Select the BEST answer in each case.

37. When a phlebotomist chooses to use a syringe in the collection of multiple blood assays from a patient, blood for which of the following assays should be delivered first?

   (A) creatinine
   (B) glucose
   (C) prothrombin time
   (D) blood urea nitrogen

38. Which of the following blood analytes has a rise and fall in values with the time of day and, thus, must be collected on time?

   (A) blood urea nitrogen
   (B) cortisol

(C) hemoglobin
(D) hematocrit

39. Therapeutic phlebotomy is used in the treatment of

(A) iron deficiency anemia
(B) chronic anemia
(C) megaloblastic anemia
(D) polycythemia

40. For the brief physical examination required to determine if the blood donor is in generally good health, the oral temperature of the blood donor must not exceed

(A) 36°C
(B) 37.5°C
(C) 38.5°C
(D) 39.5°C

41. For the brief physical examination required to determine if the blood donor is in generally good health, the donor's systolic blood pressure should measure

(A) 50 to 110 mm Hg
(B) 60 to 110 mm Hg
(C) 90 to 180 mm Hg
(D) 100 to 190 mm Hg

42. Skin tests are used to determine if a patient has ever had contact with

(A) a particular antibody and has produced antigens to that antibody
(B) a particular antigen and has produced antibodies to that antigen
(C) the disease leukemia
(D) the disease polycythemia

43. Normally, after an adult patient has ingested the 100 g of glucose in the glucose tolerance test, the glucose level should return to normal within

(A) 30 minutes after ingesting the glucose
(B) 60 minutes after ingesting the glucose
(C) 120 minutes after ingesting the glucose
(D) 180 minutes after ingesting the glucose

DIRECTIONS: For each of the questions or incomplete statements below, ONE or MORE of the numbered responses are correct. In each case select

    A. if only 1, 2, and 3 are correct
    B. if only 1 and 3 are correct
    C. if only 2 and 4 are correct
    D. if only 4 is correct
    E. if all are correct

44. Which of the following guidelines must be adhered to by the patient to properly prepare himself or herself for the GTT test?

    (1) the patient's carbohydrate intake must not exceed 20 g per day for 3 days before the GTT
    (2) the patient must not eat anything for 12 hours before the GTT but should not fast for more than 16 hours before the test
    (3) the patient should take corticosteroids 2 days before the GTT
    (4) the patient should not exercise for 12 hours before the GTT

45. Which of the following medications might interfere with the GTT test?

    (1) clofibrate
    (2) corticosteroids
    (3) estrogens
    (4) diuretics

46. Which of the following condition(s) should be reported by the patient to his or her physician before the GTT test, since the condition(s) may affect the results of the GTT test?

    (1) hyperthyroidism
    (2) pregnancy
    (3) adrenal insufficiency
    (4) acute pancreatitis

47. In the D-xylose tolerance test, what type(s) of body samples is/are analyzed for D-xylose?

    (1) blood
    (2) CSF
    (3) pooled sample of urine
    (4) random urine sample

48. Fasting blood specimens is/are usually required for determination of

    (1) glucose
    (2) cholesterol

    (3) triglycerides
    (4) hematocrit

49. Which of the following items usually is/are kept on file on every blood donor for a minimum of 5 years?

    (1) age
    (2) date of birth
    (3) a record of reason for deferrals
    (4) written consent form signed by the donor

50. For blood donor collections, the phlebotomist must always check the possible blood donor on which of the following items before the blood donation?

    (1) blood glucose value or urine glucose value
    (2) hematocrit or hemoglobin
    (3) WBC count
    (4) temperature

DIRECTIONS: Indicate whether each statement is TRUE or FALSE.

51. **True/False:** Figure 5–2 shows the correct order of draw for both the evacuated tube method and the syringe deposit method.

Evacuated tube method

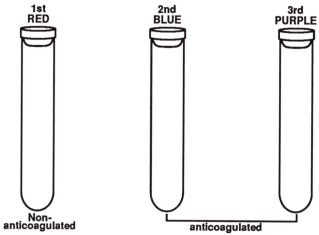

1st
RED

2nd
BLUE

3rd
PURPLE

Non-
anticoagulated

anticoagulated

Syringe deposit method

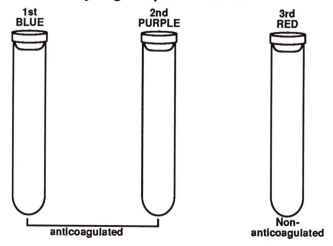

1st
BLUE

2nd
PURPLE

3rd
RED

anticoagulated

Non-
anticoagulated

Figure 5—2.

52. **True/False:** Generally, if the evacuated collection tube is held completely vertically during blood collection, transfer of anticoagulants from tube to tube will be minimal.

53. **True/False:** When a phlebotomist chooses to use a syringe for multiple blood assays, the blood should be delivered first aseptically into blood culture tubes, then into anticoagulated tubes, and finally into the tubes without anticoagulants.

54. **True/False:** A 30-mL syringe is the largest syringe recommended to draw blood specimens through central venous catheter lines.

55. **True/False:** For the D-xylose tolerance test, usually a 2-hour blood sample is taken, and a pooled sample of urine is taken over the 5-hour period after dose administration.

56. **True/False:** D-xylose is a protein found in certain fruits, such as plums, but does not normally occur in the blood or urine.

57. **True/False:** To perform a skin test, the phlebotomist should slip the needle just under the skin of the patient's forearm, and the plunger should be pulled back to ensure that a blood vessel has been entered.

58. **True/False:** For the Surgicutt bleeding time test, a Velcro tourniquet is required for the assay to be performed.

DIRECTIONS: Each of the questions or incomplete statements below is followed by suggested answers or completions. Select the BEST answer in each case.

59. For the Surgicutt bleeding time test, the blood pressure cuff must be inflated on the patient's upper arm to

    (A) 20 mm Hg
    (B) 30 mm Hg
    (C) 40 mm Hg
    (D) 60 mm Hg

60. Throat cultures most commonly are obtained to determine the presence of

    (A) *Neisseria* infection
    (B) *Streptococcus* infection
    (C) *Staphylococcus* infection
    (D) *Bacillus* infection

61. In phlebotomy, the abbreviation CVC refers to

    (A) central venous catheter
    (B) control venous catheter

(C) central venous chloride

(D) control venous chloride

62. For the sweat chloride test to be performed on a child, the best site is the

(A) arm

(B) hand

(C) leg

(D) finger

63. What is the usual dose of D-xylose administered to the patient in the D-xylose tolerance test?

(A) 10 g

(B) 25 g

(C) 75 g

(D) 100 g

64. To draw through central venous catheters, when is it permissible for the phlebotomist to disconnect an infusor or autosyringe pump?

(A) immediately before collecting the required blood

(B) immediately after collecting the required blood

(C) immediately after the second blood tube is drawn

(D) at no time is it permissible for the phlebotomist to disconnect an infusor or autosyringe pump

65. To help minimize the incidence of dizziness, fainting, or other reactions to blood loss, blood donors are encouraged to eat within

(A) 9 hours of donating blood

(B) 8 hours of donating blood

(C) 7 hours of donating blood

(D) 6 hours of donating blood

DIRECTIONS: Each group of lettered words or phrases below is followed by a list of numbered words or phrases. MATCH the lettered word or phrase most closely associated with the numbered word or phrase.

Questions 66 through 70

A. 150 g of carbohydrate per day for 3 days before the test

B. indocyanine green dye

C. epinephrine injection

66. Used to test liver function

67. Sweat chloride test

68. Glucose tolerance test

69. Gastric analysis test

D. four cups and lids with gauze pads used in procedure

E. stimulation from histamine or pentagastrin

70. Used to determine availability and quantity of liver glycogen

Questions 71 through 75

A. AABB
B. CVC
C. EDTA
D. STAT
E. BSP

71. Immediately
72. Ethylenediaminetetraacetate
73. American Association of Blood Banks
74. Bromsulphalein
75. Central venous catheter line

Questions 76 through 80

A. syringe collection
B. fasting specimen
C. peak and trough level
D. evacuated tube collection system
E. central venous catheter

76. Any tube that has an anticoagulant in it should be drawn last so that it can be mixed as soon after collection as possible

77. Very important in the collection of glucose

78. Lumen(s) not being drawn should be clamped

79. Therapeutic drug monitoring

80. The sodium citrate tube should be drawn first, followed by other anti-coagulated tubes

DIRECTIONS: Indicate whether each statement is TRUE or FALSE.

81. **True/False:** To draw blood through a CVC, the patient should be positioned by elevating the bed to have the patient sit upright, with the catheter above the level of the patient's heart.

82. **True/False:** To collect blood for a blood donation, the arm is cleansed with 70% isopropanol, and the needle is inserted into the antecubital vein.

83. **True/False:** For a blood donation, the proper amount of blood collected is between 405 and 495 mL.

84. **True/False:** The 2-hour postprandial blood specimens are drawn for glucose determinations.

85. **True/False:** Patients with cystic fibrosis produce calcium in their sweat at two to five times the level produced by healthy individuals.

86. **True/False:** In the lactose tolerance test, after lactose is given to the patient, 1-hour, 2-hour, and 3-hour blood samples are drawn and tested for lactose.

87. **True/False:** Epinephrine increases blood sugar by accelerating glycogenolysis.

88. **True/False:** The D-xylose absorption test commonly is used for the diagnosis of diabetes mellitus.

DIRECTIONS: For each of the questions or incomplete statements below, ONE or MORE of the numbered responses are correct. In each case select

    A. if only 1, 2, and 3 are correct
    B. if only 1 and 3 are correct
    C. if only 2 and 4 are correct
    D. if only 4 is correct
    E. if all are correct

89. Which of the following is/are true concerning tolerance tests?

    (1) the epinephrine tolerance test is used to determine availability and quantity of liver glycogen
    (2) the glucagon tolerance test measures glucagon levels in the blood
    (3) the lactose tolerance test measures glucose levels in the blood after lactose is administered
    (4) the D-xylose tolerance test is used commonly for the diagnosis of cystic fibrosis

90. Which of the following is/are true concerning cystic fibrosis?

    (1) indocyanine green is used in the diagnosis of cystic fibrosis
    (2) cystic fibrosis affects the lungs, upper respiratory tract, liver, and pancreas
    (3) the gastric acid secretion is tested for in the diagnosis of cystic fibrosis
    (4) pilocarpine hydrochloric acid is used in the procedure to test for cystic fibrosis

91. Figure 5–3 shows swabbing of the arm in concentric circles for preparation of drawing blood for

    (1) therapeutic drug monitoring
    (2) blood cultures

(3) lactose tolerance test
(4) blood donation

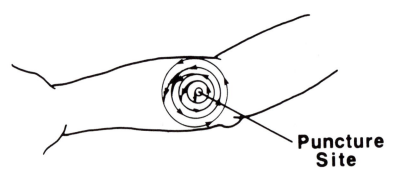

**Puncture
Site**

Figure 5–3. *From Garza, D., and Becan-McBride, K.* Phlebotomy Handbook, second edition. *Appleton & Lange: Norwalk, Ct; 1989.*

92. Nasopharyngeal cultures often are performed to detect carrier states of

    (1) *Neisseria meningitidis*
    (2) *Corynebacterium diphtheriae*
    (3) *Streptococcus pyogenes*
    (4) *Haemophilus influenzae*

93. Which of the following can lead to errors in the collection of blood for blood cultures?

    (1) palpation of the venipuncture site after the site has been prepared without first cleaning the gloved finger
    (2) injection of air into the anaerobe bottle
    (3) inoculating the anaerobe bottle last
    (4) wiping the iodine from the tops of the bottle with alcohol

94. Which of the following materials and supplies is/are needed for the Surgicutt procedure?

    (1) blood pressure cuff
    (2) butterfly-type bandage
    (3) disposable gloves
    (4) vacuum blood collection tube with EDTA

95. Which of the following methods is/are bleeding time test(s)?

    (1) Duke assay
    (2) Surgicutt assay
    (3) Ivy assay
    (4) xylose assay

96. Which of the following is/are considered timed blood specimens?

    (1) cortisol
    (2) GTT
    (3) therapeutic drug monitoring
    (4) creatinine

97. In the collection of blood for blood gases, the blood gas assay includes testing for

    (1) pH
    (2) Po_2
    (3) Pco_2
    (4) pH_2O

98. Which of the following is/are coagulopathies?

    (1) von Willebrand's disease
    (2) von Gierke's disease
    (3) thrombocytopenia
    (4) diabetes mellitus

DIRECTIONS: Each group of lettered words or phrases below is followed by a list of numbered words or phrases. MATCH the lettered word or phrase most closely associated with the numbered word or phrase.

Questions 99 through 103

A. collect blood cultures first, anti-coagulated tubes, then tubes without anticoagulants
B. diagnosis of liver dysfunction
C. collect tubes without anti-coagulants and then anti-coagulated tubes
D. treatment of myeloproliferative diseases
E. diagnostic test for glycogen stores

99. Therapeutic phlebotomy
100. Glucagon tolerance test
101. Syringe collection procedure
102. Cardiogreen dye test
103. Evacuated tube collection system

Questions 104 through 108

A. reflectance meter that measures color change

B. drawn on individuals between 17 and 66 years old

C. patient should not eat plums before test

D. patient has incision in forearm

E. patient has arterial blood drawn

104. D-xylose tolerance test
105. Blood gases
106. Rapid method for glucose determination
107. Blood donation
108. Bleeding time test

DIRECTIONS: Indicate whether each statement is TRUE or FALSE.

109. **True/False:** Dextran, strepokinase, or ethyl alcohol may cause the bleeding time to be shortened.

110. **True/False:** In the collection of blood cultures, the anaerobe bottle must be inoculated first.

111. **True/False:** In the health care setting, if someone refers to the ER, he or she is indicating the energizing radiation in radiology.

112. **True/False:** The presence of mild skin disorders, such as psoriasis, acne, or poison ivy rash, does not necessarily prohibit an individual from donating blood unless there are lesions in the antecubital area or the rash is particularly extensive.

113. **True/False:** As long as the blood bank records can trace the packed red blood cell component from a donor to its disposition, it is not necessary to trace the other components (i.e., white blood cells, platelets) to their disposition.

114. **True/False:** In order to donate blood, the donor's pulse rate must be a regular, strong pulse rate between 50 and 100 beats/minute.

115. **True/False:** If a patient is found not to be fasting when the phlebotomist arrives to collect blood for a fasting specimen, the phlebotomist should consult with the physician to determine if a nonfasting level will be of any benefit.

DIRECTIONS: Each of the questions or incomplete statements below is followed by suggested answers or completions. Select the BEST answer in each case.

116. The phlebotomist's thumb should not be used for palpating arteries in the arterial puncture procedure because the phlebotomist's thumb

(A) is usually dirty

(B) has less sensitivity than the other fingers

(C) has a pulse that may be confused with the patient's pulse
(D) has more neurons for touching, which interferes in the process of finding the patient's pulse

117. The Surgicutt bleeding time test has replaced the Duke bleeding time test because the

(A) Duke bleeding time test was too difficult to perform
(B) Surgicutt bleeding time test provides a standardized instrument for the assay
(C) Surgicutt bleeding time test takes considerably less time than the Duke bleeding time test
(D) Duke bleeding time test was too expensive in this cost-containment era of health care

118. If the patient's bleeding time is longer than the normal limits, this result may indicate the need for which of the following laboratory tests?

(A) alkaline phosphatase level
(B) acid phosphatase level
(C) platelet count
(D) blood urea nitrogen result

119. Which of the following procedures is best to help reduce the potential scarring by the Surgicutt bleeding time test?

(A) apply a butterfly-type bandage to the site of incision
(B) provide a small stitch to the site of incision
(C) apply a gauze and tape to the site of incision
(D) apply a small piece of moleskin to the site of incision

120. Which of the following procedures requires 10 mL normal saline and two or three 20-mL disposable syringes?

(A) sweat chloride procedure
(B) skin test for allergies
(C) collecting blood from a blood donor
(D) collecting blood through CVCs

121. Which of the following procedures requires blood collection for trough and peak levels?

(A) skin test for allergies
(B) therapeutic drug monitoring

(C) collecting blood through CVCs

(D) sweat chloride procedure

122. Which of the following is an excellent indicator of small intestine absorption as it passes unchanged through the liver and is excreted by the kidneys?

(A) D-xylose

(B) cardiogreen dye

(C) bromsulphalein dye

(D) indocyanine green dye

123. Which of the following tests requires passing a tube through the patient's nose and into the stomach?

(A) sweat chloride by iontophoresis

(B) Hollander test

(C) cardiogreen dye test

(D) D-xylose tolerance test

124. Which of the following procedures requires that a 3-hour glucose tolerance test be performed on the patient 1 day in advance of this procedure to determine if the patient has a normal glucose curve?

(A) D-xylose tolerance test

(B) epinephrine tolerance test

(C) glucagon tolerance test

(D) lactose tolerance test

125. Which of the following procedures is run to test the efficiency of the patient's insulin-releasing mechanism?

(A) epinephrine tolerance test

(B) glucose tolerance test

(C) glucagon tolerance test

(D) lactose tolerance test

126. Figure 5–4 illustrates a part of which of the following procedures?

(A) Lee-White clotting time

(B) cardiogreen dye test

(C) Surgicutt bleeding time test

(D) blood culture procedure

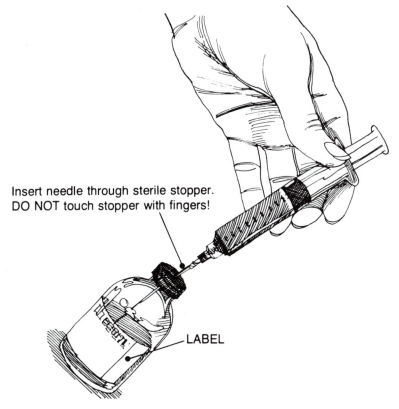

Insert needle through sterile stopper.
DO NOT touch stopper with fingers!

LABEL

Figure 5—4. *(Courtesy of College of American Pathologists, Skokie, IL.)*

127.   In the arterial blood gas procedure for adults, which of the following
anticoagulants usually is added to coat the syringe barrel?

(A) EDTA
(B) heparin
(C) oxalate
(D) citrate

Answers and Explanations

1.   **D.** Arterial blood is the specimen of choice for testing the pH, Po_2,
and Pco_2 of the blood.

Garza D, Becan-McBride K. Phlebotomy Handbook. *E. Norwalk, CT: Appleton &
Lange; 1989:113.*

2. **B.** Capillary blood gases are collected from the same areas of the body as other capillary samples, such as the lateral posterior area of the heel, the great toe, or the ball of the finger.
    Garza and Becan-McBride, p 113.

3. **C.** A heparinized capillary tube with a volume of at least 100 μL should be used to collect a specimen for capillary blood gas analysis.
    Garza and Becan-McBride, p 114.

4. **B.** The femoral artery in the groin may be used for drawing blood for arterial blood gases.
    Garza and Becan-McBride, p 114.

5. **C.** No tourniquet is required to draw blood for arterial blood gases because the artery has its own strong blood pressure.
    Garza and Becan-McBride, p 115.

6. **A.** The required amount of sample for arterial blood gases collected with a syringe and needle is usually about 1 mL.
    Garza and Becan-McBride, p 115.

7. **A.** The bleeding time test is a useful tool for testing platelet plug formation in the capillaries.
    Garza and Becan-McBride, p 115.

8. **D.** The bleeding time test is performed by making a minor standardized incision in either the earlobe or forearm.
    Garza and Becan-McBride, p 115.

9. **E.** The intake of any of the following drugs can lead to a prolonged bleeding time: aspirin, mithramycin, ethyl alcohol, and dextran.
    Garza and Becan-McBride, p 117.

10. **E.** The Lee-White clotting time is poorly reproducible and insensitive to coagulation factor deficiencies. Thus, it has been largely replaced by the prothrombin time (PT) and activated partial thromboplastin time (PTT).
    Garza and Becan-McBride, p 117.

11. **A.** Disposable gloves, iodine scrub swabstick (10% povidone-iodine solution with lathering agents), and alcohol preps are some of the items needed to collect a blood culture specimen.
    Garza and Becan-McBride, p 119.

12. **C.** For the epinephrine tolerance test, blood specimens are collected from the patient at various intervals to test for blood sugar (glucose).
    Garza and Becan-McBride, p 127.

13. **D.** The sweat chloride test is used in the diagnosis of cystic fibrosis.
Garza and Becan-McBride, p 129.

14. **A.** Bromsulphalein is a dye that has been used to test liver function. Because of the possibility of an anaphylactic response, indocyanine green (cardiogreen) more recently has been the dye of choice.
Garza and Becan-McBride, p 128.

15. **A.** Blood glucose levels are determined on patients if they are having any of the following tolerance tests performed: (1) glucagon tolerance test, (2) epinephrine tolerance test, or (3) lactose tolerance test.
Garza and Becan-McBride, pp 127–128.

16. **D.** In the sweat chloride test, which is used to diagnose cystic fibrosis, pilocarpine hydrochloric acid (HCl) is iontophoresced into the skin of the patient to stimulate sweat production.
Garza and Becan-McBride, p 129.

17. **E.** Nasopharyngeal cultures may be used to diagnose whooping cough.
Garza and Becan-McBride, p 121.

18. **A.** The skin test is administered by pulling in 0.1 mL of diluted antigen into a tuberculin syringe.
Garza and Becan-McBride, p 122.

19. **B.** The epinephrine tolerance test is used to detect von Gierke's disease.
Garza and Becan-McBride, p 127.

20. **C.** The D-xylose absorption test commonly is used for the diagnosis of malabsorption diseases of the intestine.
Garza and Becan-McBride, p 128.

21. **C.** Blood cultures often are collected from patients who have fevers of unknown origin (FGO).
Garza and Becan-McBride, p 118.

22. **D.** In patients who have symptoms suggesting problems in carbohydrate metabolism, such as diabetes mellitus, the glucose tolerance test (GTT) can be an effective diagnostic tool.
Garza and Becan-McBride, p 123.

23. **E.** To adequately evaluate the appropriate dosage levels of many drugs in therapeutic drug monitoring, the collection and evaluation of specimens for trough and peak levels is necessary.
Garza and Becan-McBride, pp 130–131.

24. **A.** The Hollander test is used to determine gastric function in terms of stomach acid production.
Garza and Becan-McBride, p 129.

25. **B.** The Surgicutt (International Technidyne Corp., Edison, NJ) is an instrument used in the bleeding time test.
Garza and Becan-McBride, p 116.

26. **FALSE.** A second site blood culture that is obtained concurrently on the opposite arm is useful when the physician suspects bacteremia due to a local, internal infection. However, a second site culture is not very effective for routine blood culture orders.
Garza and Becan-McBride, p 118.

27. **TRUE.** Most blood cultures require 3 to 5 mL of blood per bottle.
Garza and Becan-McBride, p 119.

28. **TRUE.** The 2-hour postprandial glucose test can be used to screen patients for diabetes.
Garza and Becan-McBride, p 126.

29. **FALSE.** In order to donate blood, a donor must weigh at least 110 pounds (50 kg).
Garza and Becan-McBride, p 134.

30. **TRUE.** The term STAT means immediately.
Garza and Becan-McBride, p 138.

31. **FALSE.** It is recommended that blood for serum iron be drawn before other specimens collected in tubes with EDTA to avoid interference in testing the serum iron level.
Garza and Becan-McBride, p 139.

32. **FALSE.** The capillary tube and items in Figure 5–1 are used to collect capillary, not arterial, blood gases.
Garza and Becan-McBride, p 114.

33. **TRUE.** In the Surgicutt bleeding time test (International Technidyne Corp., Edison, NJ), the phlebotomist must wick the flow of blood with filter paper every 30 seconds until blood no longer stains the paper.
Garza and Becan-McBride, p 117.

34. **FALSE.** For blood donations, the hematocrit must be no less than 38% for female donors.
Garza and Becan-McBride, p 135.

35. **FALSE.** The most common requests for timed blood specimens are glucose levels drawn 2 hours after a meal.
Garza & Becan-McBride, p. 126.

36. **FALSE.** Any blood vacuum collection tube that has an anticoagulant in it should be drawn last when multiple blood assays are requested so that it can be mixed as soon after collection as possible.
Garza and Becan-McBride, p 139.

37. **C.** When a phlebotomist chooses to use a syringe in the collection of multiple blood assays from a patient, blood for coagulation studies (i.e., prothrombin time) should be delivered to the sodium citrate tube first and mixed.
Garza and Becan-McBride, p 139.

38. **B.** Certain natural hormone levels, such as cortisol, rise and fall with the time of day and, thus, must be collected on time.
Garza and Becan-McBride, p 138.

39. **D.** Therapeutic phlebotomy is used in the treatment of some myeloproliferative diseases, such as polycythemia, or other conditions in which the removal of blood benefits the patient.
Garza and Becan-McBride, p 137.

40. **B.** For the brief physical examination required to determine if the blood donor is in generally good health, the oral temperature of the blood donor must not exceed 37.5°C.
Garza and Becan-McBride, p 135.

41. **C.** For the brief physical examination required to determine if the blood donor is in generally good health, the donor's systolic blood pressure should measure 90 to 180 mm Hg. People with a systolic blood pressure out of this range should be deferred as donors.
Garza and Becan-McBride, p 135.

42. **B.** Skins test are used to determine if a patient has ever had contact with a particular antigen and has produced antibodies to that antigen.
Garza and Becan-McBride, p 122.

43. **C.** Normally, after an adult patient has ingested the 100 g of glucose in the glucose tolerance test (GTT), the glucose level should return to normal within 2 hours after ingesting the glucose.
Garza and Becan-McBride, p 123.

44. **C.** The patient needs to follow three basic guidelines to prepare for the GTT test: (1) the patient's carbohydrate intake must be at least 150 g per day for 3 days before the GTT, (2) the patient should not eat anything for 12 hours before the GTT but should not fast for more than 16 hours before the test, and (3) the patient should not exercise for 12 hours before the GTT.
Garza and Becan-McBride, p 123.

45. **E.** Clofibrate, corticosteroids, diuretics, and estrogens all can interfere with the GTT test results.
    Garza and Becan-McBride, pp 123–124.

46. **E.** Hyperthyroidism, pregnancy, adrenal insufficiency, and acute pancreatitis are conditions that may affect the results of the GTT test.
    Garza and Becan-McBride, p 125.

47. **B.** In the D-xylose tolerance test, a 2-hour blood sample is taken, and a pooled sample of urine is taken from the patient over the 5-hour period after dose administration.
    Garza and Becan-McBride, p 128.

48. **A.** Fasting blood levels of glucose, cholesterol, and triglycerides can be very important in diagnosis of patients' conditions.
    Garza and Becan-McBride, p 138.

49. **E.** Age, date of birth, a record of reason for deferrals (if any), and a written consent form signed by the donor are some of the major items kept on file on every blood donor.
    Garza and Becan-McBride, p 134.

50. **C.** The blood bank phlebotomist must check the blood donor's temperature and hematocrit or hemoglobin value before the blood donation.
    Garza and Becan-McBride, p 135.

51. **TRUE.** Figure 5–2 shows the correct order of draw for both the evacuated tube method and the syringe deposit method.
    Garza and Becan-McBride, pp 139–140.

52. **FALSE.** Generally, if the evacuated collection tube is held horizontally or slightly down during blood collection, transfer of anticoagulants from tube to tube will be minimal.
    Garza and Becan-McBride, p 139.

53. **TRUE.** When a phlebotomist chooses to use a syringe for multiple blood assays, the blood should be delivered first aseptically into blood culture tubes, then into anticoagulated tubes, and finally into the tubes without anticoagulants.
    Garza and Becan-McBride, p 139.

54. **FALSE.** A 20-mL syringe is the largest syringe recommended to draw blood specimens through central venous catheter lines.
    Garza and Becan-McBride, p 131.

55. **TRUE.** For the D-xylose tolerance test, usually a 2-hour blood sample is taken and a pooled sample of urine is taken over the 5-hour period after dose administration.
Garza and Becan-McBride, p 128.

56. **FALSE.** D-xylose is a pentose (a 5-carbon sugar) found in certain fruits, such as plums, but does not normally occur in blood or urine.
Garza and Becan-McBride, p 128.

57. **FALSE.** To perform a skin test, the phlebotomist should slip the needle just under the skin of the patient's forearm, and the plunger should be pulled back to ensure that a blood vessel has NOT been entered.
Garza and Becan-McBride, p 122.

58. **FALSE.** For the Surgicutt bleeding time test, a blood pressure cuff is required for the assay to be performed.
Garza and Becan-McBride, p 116.

59. **C.** For the Surgicutt bleeding time test, the blood pressure cuff must be inflated on the patient's upper arm to 40 mm Hg.
Garza and Becan-McBride, p 116.

60. **B.** Throat cultures most commonly are obtained to determine the presence of a streptococcal infection.
Garza and Becan-McBride, p 121.

61. **A.** In phlebotomy, the abbreviation CVC refers to central venous catheter.
Garza and Becan-McBride, p 131.

62. **C.** For the sweat chloride test to be performed on a child, the best site is a site with the largest surface area, the leg.
Garza and Becan-McBride, p 130.

63. **B.** A measured dose of 25 g of D-xylose usually is given to the patient for the D-xylose tolerance test.
Garza and Becan-McBride, p 128.

64. **D.** At no time is it permissible for a phlebotomist to disconnect or reconnect an infusor or autosyringe pump.
Garza and Becan-McBride, p 131.

65. **D.** To help minimize the incidence of dizziness, fainting, or other reactions to blood loss, blood donors are encouraged to eat within 4 to 6 hours of donating blood.
Garza and Becan-McBride, p 134.

66. **B.** Indocyanine green dye has been used to test liver function.
    Garza and Becan-McBride, p 128.

67. **D.** Four cups and lids should be preweighed with two 2-inch square gauze pads in each cup for the sweat choride test.
    Garza and Becan-McBride, p 129.

68. **A.** For 3 days before the glucose tolerance test (GTT), the patient needs to have 150 g of carbohydrate per day.
    Garza and Becan-McBride, p 124.

69. **E.** For the gastric analysis test to be performed, gastric acid secretion must be stimulated by histamine or pentagastrin.
    Garza and Becan-McBride, p 129.

70. **C.** The epinephrine tolerance test is used to determine availability and quantity of liver glycogen by stimulating an increase in blood sugar by epinephrine injection.
    Garza and Becan-McBride, p 127.

71. **D.** The term STAT means immediately and has come to indicate that a patient's medical condition suddenly has become critical and must be treated or responded to as a medical emergency.
    Garza and Becan-McBride, p 138.

72. **C.** Ethylenediaminetetraacetate is usually abbreviated as EDTA and is a chelating anticoagulant used to collect blood specimens.
    Garza and Becan-McBride, p 139.

73. **A.** AABB stands for American Association of Blood Banks.
    Garza and Becan-McBride, p 133.

74. **E.** Bromsulphalein is sometimes abbreviated as BSP.
    Garza and Becan-McBride, p 128.

75. **B.** Blood specimens occasionally are drawn through central venous catheter lines (CVCs).
    Garza and Becan-McBride, p 131.

76. **D.** To draw blood by the evacuated tube collection system, any tube that has an anticoagulant in it should be drawn last so that it can be mixed as soon after collection as possible.
    Garza and Becan-McBride, p 139.

77. **B.** Fasting levels of glucose are very important in diagnosis.
    Garza and Becan-McBride, p 138.

78. **E.** When drawing blood from a multilumen central venous catheter, the lumens not being drawn should be clamped during the procedure to prevent dilution of the blood sample being drawn.
    Garza and Becan-McBride, p 131.

79. **C.** Laboratory drug monitoring of therapeutic agents requires the collection and evaluation of specimens for trough and peak levels.
    Garza and Becan-McBride, pp 130–131.

80. **A.** When a phlebotomist chooses to use a syringe, the order of delivery of blood to the tubes should be (1) blood is delivered to the sodium citrate tube first and mixed, and (2) blood is delivered to any other anticoagulated tube and mixed.
    Garza and Becan-McBride, p 139.

81. **FALSE.** To draw blood through a CVC, the patient should be positioned by making the bed flat, or have the catheter hub at or below the level of the patient's heart.
    Garza and Becan-McBride, p 132.

82. **FALSE.** To collect blood for a blood donation, the venipuncture site must be scrubbed with an iodine scrub swabstick.
    Garza and Becan-McBride, p 136.

83. **TRUE.** The proper amount of blood for a blood donation is between 405 and 495 mL.
    Garza and Becan-McBride, p 136.

84. **TRUE.** The 2-hour postprandial blood specimens are drawn to determine glucose levels, which are used to screen patients for diabetes.
    Garza and Becan-McBride, p 126.

85. **FALSE.** Patients with cystic fibrosis produce chloride in their sweat at two to five times the level produced by healthy individuals.
    Garza and Becan-McBride, p 129.

86. **FALSE.** In the lactose tolerance test, after lactose is given to the patient, 1-hour, 2-hour, and 3-hour blood samples are drawn and tested for glucose.
    Garza and Becan-McBride, p 128.

87. **TRUE.** Epinephrine increases blood sugar by accelerating glycogenolysis (breakdown of glycogen).
    Garza and Becan-McBride, p 127.

88. **FALSE.** The D-xylose absorption test is used for the diagnosis of malabsorption states.
    Garza and Becan-McBride, p 128.

89. **B.** The epinephrine tolerance test is used to determine availability and quantity of liver glycogen, and the lactose tolerance test measures glucose levels in the blood after lactose is administered to the patient.
Garza and Becan-McBride, pp 127–128.

90. **C.** Cystic fibrosis affects the lungs, upper respiratory tract, liver, and pancreas, and pilocarpine hydrochloric acid is used in the sweat chloride procedure to test for cystic fibrosis.
Garza and Becan-McBride, p 129.

91. **C.** Figure 5–3 shows swabbing of the arm in concentric circles for preparation of drawing blood for blood cultures or blood donations.
Garza and Becan-McBride, pp 119, 136.

92. **E.** Nasopharyngeal cultures often are performed to detect carrier states of *Neisseria meningitidis, Corynebacterium diphtheriae, Streptococcus pyogenes, Haemophilus influenzae,* and *Staphylococcus aureus.*
Garza and Becan-McBride, p 121.

93. **A.** The following can lead to errors in the collection of blood for blood cultures: (1) palpation of the venipuncture site after the site has been prepared without first cleaning the gloved finger, (2) injection of air into the anaerobe bottle, and (3) inoculating the anaerobe bottle last.
Garza and Becan-McBride, p 120.

94. **A.** A blood pressure cuff (sphygmomanometer), a butterfly-type bandage, and disposable gloves are needed for the Surgicutt procedure.
Garza and Becan-McBride, p 116.

95. **A.** Duke originally described the first method for the bleeding time assay, followed by Ivy, who improved the bleeding time assay. Recent advances have led to the Surgicutt bleeding time assay.
Garza and Becan-McBride, pp 115–116.

96. **A.** Cortisol, glucose tolerance test (GTT), and therapeutic drug monitoring are tests that require timed blood specimens.
Garza and Becan-McBride, pp 124, 137–138.

97. **A.** The blood gas assays include testing for pH, Po_2, and Pco_2.
Garza and Becan-McBride, p 113.

98. **B.** Von Willebrand's disease and thrombocytopenia are two coagulopathies (problems with blood clotting).
Garza and Becan-McBride, p 115.

99. **D.** Therapeutic phlebotomy is used in the treatment of some myeloproliferative diseases, such as polycythemia.
Garza and Becan-McBride, p 137.

100.   **E.** The glucagon tolerance test is conducted to test for liver glycogen storage.
Garza and Becan-McBride, p 127.

101.   **A.** For the syringe collection procedure, blood culture tubes are collected first, followed by anticoagulated tubes, then tubes without anticoagulants.
Garza and Becan-McBride, p 139.

102.   **B.** Cardiogreen (indocyanine green) dye is the dye of choice in the testing of liver function.
Garza and Becan-McBride, p 128.

103.   **C.** For the evacuated tube collection system, tubes without anticoagulants are collected, and then anticoagulated tubes are collected.
Garza and Becan-McBride, p 139.

104.   **C.** For the D-xylose tolerance test, the patient should not eat plums for up to 3 days before the test because plums have D-xylose, which will interfere in the test procedure.
Garza and Becan-McBride, p 128.

105.   **E.** Adult patients usually have arterial blood collected for blood gases.
Garza and Becan-McBride, pp 114–115.

106.   **A.** Many of the rapid methods for glucose testing use a reflectance meter, which measures color change as glucose in the patient's specimen reacts with reagents on a dipstick pad.
Garza and Becan-McBride, p 126.

107.   **B.** In order to donate blood, a donor should be between the ages of 17 and 66 years.
Garza and Becan-McBride, p 134.

108.   **D.** The bleeding time test is performed by making a minor standardized incision in either the earlobe or forearm.
Garza and Becan-McBride, p 115.

109.   **FALSE.** Dextran, streptokinase, or ethyl alcohol may cause a prolonged bleeding time.
Garza and Becan-McBride, p 117.

110.   **TRUE.** In the collection of blood cultures, the anaerobe bottle must be inoculated first.
Garza and Becan-McBride, p 120.

111. **FALSE.** In the health care setting, someone referring to the ER is indicating the emergency room.
Garza and Becan-McBride, p 141.

112. **TRUE.** The presence of mild skin disorders, such as psoriasis, acne, or poison ivy rash, does not necessarily prohibit an individual from donating blood unless there are lesions in the antecubital area or the rash is particularly extensive.
Garza and Becan-McBride, p 135.

113. **FALSE.** The blood bank records must be able to trace all components of a donor unit (e.g., red blood cells, white blood cells, platelets) to their disposition.
Garza and Becan-McBride, p 134.

114. **TRUE.** In order to donate blood, the donor's pulse rate must be a regular, strong pulse rate between 50 and 100 beats/minute.
Garza and Becan-McBride, p 135.

115. **TRUE.** If a patient is found not to be fasting when the phlebotomist arrives to collect blood for a fasting specimen, the phlebotomist should consult with the physician to determine if a nonfasting level will be of any benefit.
Garza and Becan-McBride, p 138.

116. **C.** The phlebotomist's thumb should not be used for palpating arteries in the arterial puncture procedure because there is a pulse in the thumb that may be confused with the patient's pulse.
Garza and Becan-McBride, p 115.

117. **B.** The Surgicutt bleeding time test has replaced the Duke bleeding time test because the Surgicutt bleeding time test provides a standardized instrument for the assay.
Garza and Becan-McBride, pp 115–116.

118. **C.** A prolonged bleeding time may indicate the need for further coagulation testing, such as the platelet count.
Garza and Becan-McBride, p 117.

119. **A.** Applying butterfly-type bandages to the incision area for a 24-hour period can reduce the potential scarring from a Surgicutt bleeding time instrument.
Garza and Becan-McBride, p 116.

120. **D.** Two or three 20-mL disposable syringes and 10 mL normal saline for flushing the catheter are needed to collect blood through central venous catheter lines (CVCs).
Garza and Becan-McBride, p 131.

121. **B.** To adequately evaluate the appropriate dosage level of many drugs, the collection and evaluation of specimens for trough and peak levels is necessary in therapeutic drug monitoring.
      Garza and Becan-McBride, pp 130–131.

122. **A.** D-xylose is an excellent indicator of small intestine absorption as it passes unchanged through the liver and is excreted by the kidneys.
      Garza and Becan-McBride, p 128.

123. **B.** The Hollander test involves passing a tube through the patient's nose and into the stomach.
      Garza and Becan-McBride, p 129.

124. **D.** The lactose tolerance test requires that a 3-hour glucose tolerance test be performed 1 day in advance to determine if the patient has a normal glucose tolerance curve.
      Garza and Becan-McBride, p 128.

125. **B.** The glucose tolerance test is run to test the efficiency of the patient's insulin-releasing mechanism.
      Garza and Becan-McBride, p 123.

126. **D.** Figure 5–4 illustrates the inoculation of a blood culture bottle in the blood culture procedure.
      Garza and Becan-McBride, pp 119–120.

127. **B.** In the arterial blood gas procedure for adults, the addition of a small amount of liquid heparin to coat the syringe barrel will anticoagulate the blood.
      Garza and Becan-McBride, p 115.

CHAPTER 6

Infection Control and Equipment Safety

Questions

DIRECTIONS: Each of the questions or incomplete statements below is followed by suggested answers or completions. Select the BEST answer in each case.

1. Which of the following is a commonly identified pathogenic microorganism causing a skin nosocomial infection?

   (A) *Candida albicans*
   (B) *Haemophilus influenzae*
   (C) *Haemophilus vaginalis*
   (D) *Moraxella lacunata*

2. A nosocomial infection will occur when

   (A) a source is detected
   (B) the chain of infection is complete
   (C) means of transmission is maintained by disinfectants
   (D) a susceptible host remains stable

3. Which of the following infections usually has a 40% prevalence rate for nosocomial infections?

   (A) bacteremia
   (B) wound infections
   (C) respiratory infections
   (D) urinary tract infections

4. Which of the following is a commonly identified causative agent of a nosocomial infection in the nursery unit?

   (A) *Escherichia coli*
   (B) *Haemophilus vaginalis* gardnerella

(C) *Shigella* sp.
(D) *Vibrio cholerae*

5. Which of the following chemical compounds is an antiseptic for skin?

(A) 1% phenol
(B) hexachlorophene
(C) chlorophenol
(D) ethylene oxide

6. Which of the following statements is true? Disinfectants

(A) are chemicals used to inhibit the growth and development of microorganisms but not necessarily kill them
(B) are used frequently on skin
(C) are chemicals used to remove or kill pathogenic microorganisms
(D) are quaternary ammonium compounds

7. HIV is an abbreviation for

(A) hepatitis internal virus
(B) human infected virus
(C) hepatitis immunodeficiency virus
(D) human immunodeficiency virus

8. Which of the following is a commonly occurring pathogenic agent causing nosocomial infections of the gastrointestinal tract?

(A) *Neisseria gonorrhoeae*
(B) *Vibrio cholerae*
(C) *Haemophilus vaginalis*
(D) *Bordetella pertussis*

9. Which of the following types of isolation frequently is required for patients with infections that are transmitted by ingestion of a pathogen?

(A) respiratory isolation
(B) skin isolation
(C) enteric isolation
(D) reverse isolation

DIRECTIONS: For each of the questions or incomplete statements below, ONE or MORE of the numbered responses are correct. In each case select

  A. if only 1, 2, and 3 are correct
  B. if only 1 and 3 are correct
  C. if only 2 and 4 are correct

D. if only 4 is correct
E. if all are correct

10. Which of the following is/are an antiseptic for skin?

    (1) ethyl alcohol
    (2) isopropyl alcohol
    (3) chlorohexidine
    (4) hexylresorcinol

11. An employee of a health care institution with which of the following diseases must avoid patient contact by not working until the disease has healed?

    (1) hepatitis B
    (2) impetigo
    (3) chickenpox
    (4) rubella

12. Which of the following is/are commonly identified pathogenic microorganism(s) causing a nosocomial infection of the ear?

    (1) *Pseudomonas aeruginosa*
    (2) *Streptococcus pneumoniae*
    (3) gram-negative bacilli
    (4) *Moraxella lacunata*

13. Which of the following disease(s) usually will lead to strict or complete isolation?

    (1) anthrax
    (2) *Vibrio* infection
    (3) rabies
    (4) *Salmonella* infection

14. Which of the following patients is/are placed in protective or reverse isolation? Patients

    (1) with combined immunodeficiencies
    (2) with *Escherichia coli* infection
    (3) in burn units
    (4) having tuberculosis

15. In which of the following ways does the clinical laboratory contribute to infection control programs?

    (1) maintenance of laboratory records for surveillance purposes
    (2) reporting of infectious agents, drug-resistant microorganisms, and outbreaks

(3) evaluating the effectiveness of sterilization or decontamination procedures

(4) maintenance of nursing records for surveillance of medication rates

DIRECTIONS: Each group of lettered words or phrases below is followed by a list of numbered words or phrases. MATCH the lettered word or phrase most closely associated with the numbered word or phrase.

Questions 16 through 20

A. hydrogen peroxide
B. *Yersinia enterocoliticus*
C. *Streptococcus pyogenes*
D. *Haemophilus vaginalis*
E. glutaraldehyde

16. Gastrointestinal tract pathogenic agent in nosocomial infections
17. Genital tract pathogenic agent in nosocomial infections
18. Disinfectant (toxic)
19. Respiratory tract pathogenic agent in nosocomial infections
20. Antiseptic for skin

Questions 21 through 25

A. ingredient in many soaps
B. iodine
C. chlorine
D. alcohol
E. phenolic compound

21. Hypochlorite solutions
22. Quaternary ammonium compounds
23. Ethanol
24. Chlorohexidine
25. Tincture

DIRECTIONS: Indicate whether each statement is TRUE or FALSE.

26. **True/False:** Strict handwashing procedure must be adhered to for infection control in a burn unit, but gowning, gloving, and double-bagging are not used.
27. **True/False:** Microscopic airborne droplets may carry infectious agents, such as the causative agents of tuberculosis and Legionnaire's disease.
28. **True/False:** Toys are not considered a potential mode of transmitting nosocomial infections.
29. **True/False:** A phlebotomist having strep throat is not considered infectious to patients, and thus he or she may continue working while infected with the group A *Streptococcus*.
30. **True/False:** All microorganisms are considered pathogenic agents

that can cause nosocomial infections in the intensive care or postoperative unit.

31. **True/False:** For respiratory isolation, the phlebotomist must wear a mask when entering the patient's room.

32. **True/False:** The isolation technique for laboratory personnel requires no handwashing, since disposable gloves must be worn in the procedure.

DIRECTIONS: For each of the questions or incomplete statements below, ONE or MORE of the numbered responses are correct. In each case select

   A. if only 1, 2, and 3 are correct
   B. if only 1 and 3 are correct
   C. if only 2 and 4 are correct
   D. if only 4 is correct
   E. if all are correct

33. Which of the following is/are considered vector(s) in transmitting infectious diseases?

   (1) age
   (2) mosquitoes
   (3) rabies
   (4) mites

34. Which of the following can make a patient a potential host for a nosocomial infection?

   (1) chemotherapy
   (2) cancer
   (3) antibiotics
   (4) acquired immunodeficiency syndrome (AIDS)

35. Which of the following make up the chain of infection that leads to nosocomial infections?

   (1) source
   (2) mode of transmission
   (3) susceptible host
   (4) susceptible vector

36. Babies whose mothers have which of the following problems must be isolated from other infants? The mother has

   (1) been burned
   (2) cancer

(3) kidney failure and is in a dialysis unit

(4) genital herpes

37. Good technique in handwashing for the prevention of disease transmission in hospitals involve(s)

(1) warm running water

(2) soap

(3) friction

(4) hand lotion or oil

38. The actual occurrence of an infection from a biohazardous specimen depends on the

(1) virulence of the host

(2) virulence of the infecting agent

(3) susceptibility of the infecting agent

(4) susceptibility of the host

39. Which of the following can lead to a laboratory-acquired infection?

(1) drinking a coke in the specimen collection area

(2) popping the cap off a vacuum blood collection tube

(3) scratches from a needle

(4) rubbing one's eyes

DIRECTIONS: Each group of lettered words or phrases below is followed by a list of numbered words or phrases. MATCH the lettered word or phrase most closely associated with the numbered word or phrase.

Questions 40 through 44

A. interrupts the chain of infection between the source and susceptible host

B. interrupts the chain of infection between mode of transmission and susceptible host

C. interrupts the chain of infection between source and mode of transmission

D. factor that affects the host susceptibility

E. vector in transmitting infectious diseases

40. Tick

41. Limiting use of common facilities

42. Immunizations

43. Housekeeping

44. Drugs

Question 45 through 49

A. trash, linens, and other articles in an isolation room must be removed in this manner
B. the first and last step of any isolation procedure
C. should be pulled over ends of gown sleeves
D. should be tied in two places but becomes ineffective after prolonged use
E. should be large enough to cover all clothing

45. Gowning
46. Masking
47. Double-bagging
48. Handwashing
49. Gloving

DIRECTIONS: Indicate whether each statement is TRUE or FALSE.

50. True/False: Virulent organisms can enter through conjunctiva of the eye.
51. True/False: Rubbing the patient's skin with an alcohol pad destroys all microorganisms.
52. True/False: As a matter of general patient safety, it is important for the phlebotomist to empty full ashtrays in the trash can for the patient.
53. True/False: If blood is backing up the IV line from the needle insertion to the IV drip container, the IV line is working effectively.
54. True/False: When exiting an isolation room, the phlebotomist should remove the mask by carefully untying the lower tie first and then the upper one.
55. True/False: In accordance with the universal precautions for hepatitis and human immunodeficiency virus (HIV), it is extremely important to recap needles after they are used.
56. True/False: Laboratorians have a lower incidence of hepatitis antigen, tuberculosis, tularemia, and Rocky Mountain spotted fever than other hospital personnel.
57. True/False: For infection control in a burn unit, all supplies and equipment are maintained outside the plastic curtain surrounding the patient's bed.
58. True/False: As shown in Figure 6–1, source, mode of transmission, and susceptible host are the three necessary components referred to as the chain of command.

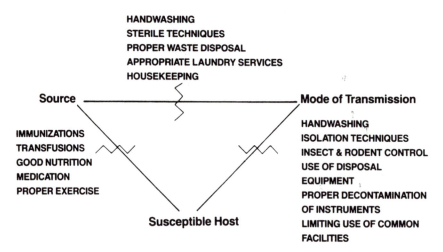

HANDWASHING
STERILE TECHNIQUES
PROPER WASTE DISPOSAL
APPROPRIATE LAUNDRY SERVICES
HOUSEKEEPING

Source ——————————————— Mode of Transmission

IMMUNIZATIONS
TRANSFUSIONS
GOOD NUTRITION
MEDICATION
PROPER EXERCISE

HANDWASHING
ISOLATION TECHNIQUES
INSECT & RODENT CONTROL
USE OF DISPOSAL
EQUIPMENT
PROPER DECONTAMINATION
OF INSTRUMENTS
LIMITING USE OF COMMON
FACILITIES

Susceptible Host

Figure 6–1. *From Garza, D., and Becan-McBride, K.* Phlebotomy Handbook, *second edition.* Norwalk, Ct: Appleton & Lange; 1989.

DIRECTIONS: For each of the questions or incomplete statements below, ONE or MORE of the numbered responses are correct. In each case select

A. if only 1, 2, and 3 are correct
B. if only 1 and 3 are correct
C. if only 2 and 4 are correct
D. if only 4 is correct
E. if all are correct

59. Which of the following is/are infection control responsibilities of the phlebotomist?

    (1) reporting personal illnesses to supervisors
    (2) reporting potential candidates for infection control, for example, patients who are jaundiced
    (3) reporting violations of infection control policies
    (4) becoming familiar with and observing all isolation policies

60. If a phlebotomist is in her first or second trimester of pregnancy, which of the following statements is/are true? The pregnant phlebotomist

    (1) may work
    (2) should work only in the laboratory
    (3) should avoid patient contact with patients having viral or rickettsial infections or those being treated with radioactive material
    (4) should avoid all patient contact

61. If a phlebotomist has the German measles, which of the following statements is/are true? He or she

(1) may work in the laboratory area only for first 5 days of rash
(2) should take sick leave
(3) may work but should not have patient contact
(4) should not work until rash is cleared (minimum of 5 days).

62. The work status should be "off from work" for the phlebotomist if he or she has

    (1) strep throat
    (2) scabies
    (3) mononucleosis
    (4) hepatitis A

63. Which of the following body areas can have any microorganisms as commonly identified pathogenic agents causing nosocomial infections?

    (1) blood and cerebrospinal fluid
    (2) genital tract
    (3) urinary tract
    (4) ear

64. Which of the following illnesses usually is transmitted from one person to another by coughing or sneezing?

    (1) scabies
    (2) Legionnaire's disease
    (3) impetigo
    (4) tuberculosis

65. For Table 6–1A, fill in the blanks to define the chemical compound as a disinfectant or an antiseptic.

TABLE 6–1A. COMMON HOSPITAL ANTISEPTICS AND DISINFECTANTS

Ethyl alcohol	_____
Isopropyl alcohol	_____
Chloramine	_____
Hypochlorite solution	_____
Ethylene oxide	_____
Formaldehyde	_____
Glutaraldehyde	_____
Hydrogen peroxide	_____
Tincture of iodine	_____
Iodophors	_____
Mercury compounds	_____
1%–2% phenols	_____
Chlorophenol	_____
Chlorohexidine	_____
Hexachlorophene	_____
Hexylresorcinol	_____
Quaternary ammonium compounds	_____

DIRECTIONS: Each of the questions or incomplete statements below is followed by suggested answers or completions. Select the BEST answer in each case.

66. Which of the following statements is not true concerning sterile techniques for phlebotomists?

    (A) rubbing the patient's skin with an alcohol pad does not destroy all of the bacteria
    (B) chemically clean gloves are the same as sterile gloves
    (C) if a needle is used for an unsuccessful venipuncture, it must be discarded and replaced with a new one before attempting another puncture
    (D) once the covering of a needle has been removed, it should not touch anything until it punctures the skin

67. Which of the following is not considered one of the "links" in the chain of infection?

    (A) susceptible host
    (B) poor isolation technique
    (C) source
    (D) mode of transmission

68. Figure 6–2 illustrates which of the following steps in specific isolation techniques for the phlebotomist?

    (A) discarding the patient's bed linens
    (B) double-bagging
    (C) removing the phlebotomist's gown
    (D) removing the IV line that has been discarded by the phlebotomist

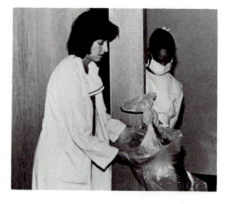

Figure 6–2. *From Garza, D., and Becan-McBride, K.* Phlebotomy Handbook, second edition. *Norwalk, Ct: Appleton & Lange; 1989.*

69. Which of the following is not a safety rule for phlebotomists to follow in patient rooms?

    (A) full ashtrays should be emptied into the trash can to avoid a fire hazard
    (B) unusual odors in the patient's room should be reported to the nursing station
    (C) phlebotomists should not touch electrical instruments located adjacent to the patient's bed
    (D) if the patient has an IV and the site is swollen and reddish, this problem should be reported to the nursing station

70. Clean (nonsterile) disposable gloves may be used for all isolation procedures except

    (A) respiratory isolation
    (B) enteric isolation
    (C) protective isolation
    (D) strict isolation

71. Which of the following illnesses can lead to enteric isolation?

    (A) mumps
    (B) measles
    (C) smallpox
    (D) amebic dysentery

72. Which of the following is not considered a factor that links the susceptible host to the source in the infectious chain?

    (A) chemotherapy
    (B) antibiotics
    (C) radiation therapy
    (D) good nutrition

73. Infection control programs aim at breaking the infection chain at one or more spots. Indicate where the items in Table 6–2A interrupt the chain of nosocomial infection.

TABLE 6–2A. CHAIN OF NOSOCOMIAL INFECTION AND HOW IT IS INTERRUPTED BY INFECTION CONTROL PROCEDURES

1. Good nutrition
2. Use of disposal equipment
3. Proper exercise
4. Immunizations
5. Limiting use of common facilities

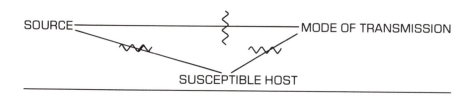

SOURCE ——————————————— MODE OF TRANSMISSION

SUSCEPTIBLE HOST

Answers and Explanations

1. **A.** *Candida albicans* is a commonly identified pathogenic agent causing skin nosocomial infections.

   Garza D, and Becan-McBride K. Phlebotomy Handbook. E. Norwalk, CT: Appleton & Lange; 1989:169. pp 148–149.

2. **B.** Nosocomial infections occur when the chain of infection is complete. The three components that make up the chain are source, means of transmission, and susceptible host.

   Garza and Becan-McBride, p 147.

3. **D.** Urinary tract infections have a prevalence rate of 40% for nosocomial infections.

   Garza and Becan-McBride, p 146.

4. **A.** *Escherichia coli* is a commonly identified pathogenic agent causing nosocomial infections in the nursery unit.

   Garza and Becan-McBride, p 148.

5. **B.** Hexachlorophene is an antiseptic for skin used frequently in surgery.

   Garza and Becan-McBride, p 165.

6. **C.** Disinfectants are chemical compounds used to remove or kill pathogenic microorganisms.

   Garza and Becan-McBride, p 165.

7. **D.** HIV is an abbreviation for human immunodeficiency virus.

   Garza and Becan-McBride, p 155.

8. **B.** *Vibrio cholerae* is a pathogenic agent that is commonly identified as a pathogenic agent in nosocomial infections of the gastrointestinal tract.
    Garza and Becan-McBride, p 148.

9. **C.** Enteric isolation frequently is required for patients with infections that are transmitted by ingestion of a pathogen.
    Garza and Becan-McBride, p 152.

10. **E.** Ethyl alcohol, isopropyl alcohol, chlorohexidine, and hexylresorcinol all are antiseptics for skin use.
    Garza and Becan-McBride, p 165.

11. **E.** If an employee of a health care institution has hepatitis B, impetigo, chickenpox, or rubella, he or she cannot work at the health care institution until the disease is noninfectious.
    Garza and Becan-McBride, p 150.

12. **A.** *Pseudomonas aeruginosa, Streptococcus pneumoniae,* and gram-negative bacilli are commonly identified pathogenic microorganisms causing a nosocomial infection of the ear.
    Garza and Becan-McBride, p 148.

13. **B.** Strict or complete isolation is required for patients with contagious diseases that may be transmitted by direct contact and via the air. Anthrax and rabies are examples leading to strict or complete isolation.
    Garza and Becan-McBride, p 152.

14. **B.** Patients with combined immunodeficiencies or in burn units are placed in protective or reverse isolation because they are highly susceptible to infection and need to be protected from the external environment.
    Garza and Becan-McBride, p 156.

15. **A.** The clinical laboratory contributes to infection control programs by (1) maintenance of laboratory records for surveillance purposes, (2) reporting of infectious agents, drug-resistant microorganisms, and outbreaks, and (3) evaluating the effectiveness of sterilization or decontamination procedures.
    Garza and Becan-McBride, p 158.

16. **B.** *Yersenia enterocoliticus* is a commonly identified pathogenic agent causing nosocomial infections in the gastrointestinal tract.
    Garza and Becan-McBride, p 148.

17. **D.** *Haemophilus vaginalis* is a commonly identified pathogenic agent causing nosocomial infection in the genital tract.
    Garza and Becan-McBride, p 148.

18. **E.** Glutaraldehyde is a toxic disinfectant.
     Garza and Becan-McBride, p 165.

19. **C.** *Streptococcus pyogenes* is a commonly identified pathogenic agent causing nosocomial infections in the respiratory tract.
     Garza and Becan-McBride, p 148.

20. **A.** Hydrogen peroxide is a commonly used antiseptic for the skin.
     Garza and Becan-McBride, p 165.

21. **C.** Hypochlorite solutions are chloride compounds used as disinfectants.
     Garza and Becan-McBride, p 165.

22. **A.** Quaternary ammonium compounds are a main ingredient in many soaps.
     Garza and Becan-McBride, p 165.

23. **D.** Ethanol is an alcohol used as an antiseptic for skin.
     Garza and Becan-McBride, p 165.

24. **E.** Chlorohexidine is a phenolic compound used as an antiseptic for skin.
     Garza and Becan-McBride, p 165.

25. **B.** Tincture is an iodine solution used as an antiseptic for skin.
     Garza and Becan-McBride, p 165.

26. **FALSE.** Strict handwashing, gowning, gloving, and double-bagging should be used for infection control in a burn unit.
     Garza and Becan-McBride, p 157.

27. **TRUE.** Microscopic airborne droplets may carry infectious agents, such as the causative agents of tuberculosis and Legionnaire's disease.
     Garza and Becan-McBride, p 149.

28. **FALSE.** Toys are a potential mode of transmission of nosocomial infections.
     Garza and Becan-McBride, p 151.

29. **FALSE.** A phlebotomist having strep throat is considered infectious to patients, and thus he or she may work only after being placed on an appropriate antibiotic and being symptom free.
     Garza and Becan-McBride, p 150.

30. **TRUE.** Any microorganisms are commonly identified pathogenic agents causing nosocomial infections in the intensive care or postoperative unit.
     Garza and Becan-McBride, p 148.

31. **TRUE.** Anyone entering a patient's room designated for respiratory isolation must wear a mask.
    Garza and Becan-McBride, p 152.

32. **FALSE.** The isolation technique for laboratory personnel requires handwashing and the wearing of disposable gloves.
    Garza and Becan-McBride, p 154.

33. **C.** Mosquitoes and mites act as vectors is transmitting infectious diseases.
    Garza and Becan-McBride, p 151.

34. **E.** Chemotherapy, cancer, antibiotics, and AIDS can all change the status of the human body, making it a potential host for a nosocomial infection.
    Garza and Becan-McBride, p 151.

35. **A.** The three components that make up the chain of infection that leads to nosocomial infections are (1) source, (2) mode of transmission, and (3) susceptible host.
    Garza and Becan-McBride, p 147.

36. **D.** Babies whose mothers have genital herpes must be isolated from other infants.
    Garza and Becan-McBride, p 157.

37. **A.** Good technique in handwashing for the prevention of disease transmission in hospitals involves warm running water, soap, and friction.
    Garza and Becan-McBride, p 159.

38. **C.** The actual occurrence of an infection from a biohazardous specimen depends on the virulence of the infecting agent and the susceptibility of the host.
    Garza and Becan-McBride, p 163.

39. **E.** A laboratory-acquired infection can result from (1) drinking or eating in the specimen collection area, (2) popping the cap off a vacuum collection tube, (3) scratches acquired from a needle and (4) rubbing one's eyes.
    Garza and Becan-McBride, pp 163–164.

40. **E.** The tick can act as a vector in transmitting infectious diseases.
    Garza and Becan-McBride, p 151.

41. **B.** Limiting use of common facilities is one method to interrupt the chain of infection between mode of transmission and susceptible host.
    Garza and Becan-McBride, p 151.

42. **A.** Immunizations is one method to interrupt the chain of infection between source and susceptible host.
     Garza and Becan-McBride, p 151.

43. **C.** Housekeeping is a method to interrupt the chain of infection between source and mode of transmission.
     Garza and Becan-McBride, p 151.

44. **D.** Drugs are a factor that affects host susceptibility to a nosocomial infection.
     Garza and Becan-McBride, p 151.

45. **E.** Gowning for isolation procedures requires a sterile gown that should be large enough to cover all clothing.
     Garza and Becan-McBride, p 162.

46. **D.** Masks should be tied in two places but become ineffective after prolonged use.
     Garza and Becan-McBride, pp 159–162.

47. **A.** Trash, linens, and other articles in an isolation room must be removed by using the double-bagging procedure.
     Garza and Becan-McBride, p 163.

48. **B.** Handwashing is the first and last step of any isolation procedure.
     Garza and Becan-McBride, p 159.

49. **C.** Gloving for isolation procedures requires the gloves to be pulled over the ends of the gown sleeves.
     Garza and Becan-McBride, p 162.

50. **TRUE.** Virulent organisms can enter through conjunctiva of the eye.
     Garza and Becan-McBride, p 163.

51. **FALSE.** Although rubbing with alcohol pads destroys most of the bacteria, it does not destroy all microorganisms.
     Garza and Becan-McBride, p 164.

52. **FALSE.** As a matter of general patient safety, it is important for the phlebotomist to empty full ashtrays in the toilet for the patient. If an ashtray is emptied in a trash can, it provides a potential fire hazard.
     Garza and Becan-McBride, p 166.

53. **FALSE.** If blood is backing up the IV line from the needle insertion to the IV drip container, the IV solution container is empty.
     Garza and Becan-McBride, p 166.

54. **TRUE.** When exiting an isolation room, the phlebotomist should remove the mask by carefully untying the lower tie first and then the upper one.
Garza and Becan-McBride, p 162.

55. **FALSE.** In accordance with the universal precautions for hepatitis and human immunodeficiency virus (HIV), it is extremely important not to recap needles after they are used. The needles should be placed in puncture-resistant containers for transport to the reprocessing area.
Garza and Becan-McBride, p 155.

56. **FALSE.** Laboratorians have a higher incidence of hepatitis antigen, tuberculosis, tularemia, and Rocky Mountain spotted fever than other hospital personnel.
Garza and Becan-McBride, p 158.

57. **TRUE.** For infection control in a burn unit, all supplies and equipment are maintained outside the plastic curtain surrounding the patient's bed.
Garza and Becan-McBride, p 157.

58. **FALSE.** Source, mode of transmission, and susceptible host make up the chain of infection.
Garza and Becan-McBride, pp 147, 151.

59. **E.** The infection control responsibilities for the phlebotomist include (1) reporting personal illnesses to supervisors, (2) reporting potential candidates for infection control, for example, patients who are jaundiced, (3) reporting violations of infection control policies, and (4) becoming familiar with and observing all isolation policies.
Garza and Becan-McBride, p 159.

60. **B.** If a phlebotomist is in her first or second trimester of pregnancy, she may work as a phlebotomist but should avoid patient contact with patients having viral or rickettsial infections and those being treated with radioactive material.
Garza and Becan-McBride, p 150.

61. **C.** If a phlebotomist has the German measles, he or she should take sick leave until the rash is cleared (minimum of 5 days).
Garza and Becan-McBride, p 150.

62. **E.** The work status should be "off from work" for the phlebotomist who has strep throat, scabies, mononucleosis, or hepatitis A.
Garza and Becan-McBride, p 150.

63. **B.** Blood, cerebrospinal fluid, and urinary tract can have any microorganisms as commonly identified pathogenic agents causing nosocomial infections.

    Garza and Becan-McBride, pp 148–149.

64. **C.** Legionnaire's disease and tuberculosis are illnesses that usually are transmitted via microscopic airborne droplets, such as when an individual coughs or sneezes, when linens are skaken, or when ventilation is not adequate.

    Garza and Becan-McBride, p 149.

65. **Table 6–1B** provides the answers.

TABLE 6–1B. COMMON HOSPITAL ANTISEPTICS AND DISINFECTANTS

Ethyl alcohol	Antiseptic
Isopropyl alcohol	Antiseptic
Chloramine	Disinfectant
Hypochlorite solution	Disinfectant
Ethylene oxide	Disinfectant
Formaldehyde	Disinfectant
Glutaraldehyde	Disinfectant
Hydrogen peroxide	Antiseptic
Tincture of iodine	Antiseptic
Iodophors	Antiseptic
Mercury compounds	Antiseptic
1%–2% Phenols	Disinfectant
Chlorophenol	Disinfectant
Chlorohexidine	Antiseptic
Hexachlorophene	Antiseptic
Hexylresorcinol	Antiseptic
Quaternary ammonium compounds	Antiseptic

66. **B.** Some manufacturers produce gloves that are chemically clean but not necessarily sterile.

    Garza and Becan-McBride, p 165.

67. **B.** The chain of infection includes (1) susceptible host, (2) source, and (3) mode of transmission.

    Garza and Becan-McBride, p 147.

68. **B.** Figure 6–2 illustrates the specific isolation technique of double-bagging that occurs after the phlebotomist has collected the blood from a patient in isolation.

    Garza and Becan-McBride, pp 161, 163.

69. **A.** To avoid a fire hazard, full ashtrays should be emptied in the toilet, never in the trash can.
Garza and Becan-McBride, p 166.

70. **C.** Sometimes, patients are placed in isolation because they are highly susceptible to infection and need to be protected from the external environment. Thus, sterile disposable gloves should be used in protective (reverse) isolation.
Garza and Becan-McBride, pp 156, 162.

71. **D.** Amebic dysentery and other parasitic infections can lead to enteric isolation.
Garza and Becan-McBride, p 152.

72. **D.** Good nutrition interrupts the chain of nosocomial infection between the susceptible host and the source.
Garza and Becan-McBride, p 151.

73. **Table 6–2B** provides the answers.

TABLE 6–2B. CHAIN OF NOSOCOMIAL INFECTION AND HOW IT IS INTERRUPTED BY INFECTION CONTROL PROCEDURES

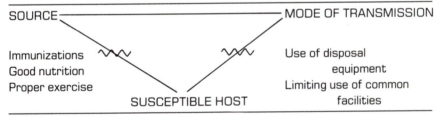

CHAPTER 7

Specimen Requisitions, Transportation, and Reporting Mechanisms

Questions

DIRECTIONS: Indicate whether each statement is TRUE or FALSE.

1. **True/False:** An effective laboratory communication network that best serves the patient includes the patient, the physician, and the laboratory personnel.
2. **True/False:** Both interlaboratory and intralaboratory communication networks are needed for effective management in a clinical laboratory.
3. **True/False:** Continuing education courses do not necessarily involve college credit.
4. **True/False:** Specimens containing viable microorganisms should be mailed using two containers.
5. **True/False:** The most error-free way to transmit laboratory requests is by personally delivering handwritten requisition forms to the laboratory.
6. **True/False:** A centralized specimen dropoff area generally reduces the problem of misplaced forms or specimens.
7. **True/False:** Bar codes help reduce transcription errors and speed up sample processing.
8. **True/False:** Bar codes are designed only for social security numbers.

DIRECTIONS: Each group of lettered words or phrases below is followed by a list of numbered words or phrases. MATCH the lettered word or phrase most closely associated with the numbered word or phrase.

Questions 9 through 12

A. quality control procedures   9. Pertain to personnel management issues

B. technical procedures

C. safety procedures

D. administrative procedures

10. Pertain to the quality of each laboratory test

11. Pertain to analytical techniques to be
followed

12. Pertain to appropriate behavior during a fire

Questions 13 through 18

A. CPU

B. ROM

C. CRT

D. RAM

E. Fortran

F. Bar code

13. Computer code that allows for rapid scanning of
numbers and letters

14. Random access memory

15. Programming language

16. Read only memory

17. Computer terminal

18. Central processing unit

**DIRECTIONS: For each of the questions or incomplete statements below,
ONE or MORE of the numbered responses are correct. In each case select**

    A. if only 1, 2, and 3 are correct
    B. if only 1 and 3 are correct
    C. if only 2 and 4 are correct
    D. if only 4 is correct
    E. if all are correct

19. Staff meetings are important for which of the following reasons?

    (1) discussing specimen collection problems
    (2) reviewing new policies
    (3) having inservices
    (4) providing a coffee break

20. In the clinical laboratory, the functions of a laboratory computer system include

    (1) entering patients' tests ordered
    (2) generating specimen collection lists for the phlebotomists
    (3) generating preprinted collection labels
    (4) sending laboratory results to the nursing station

21. When designing a blank laboratory requisition form, which of the
following factors should be considered?

    (1) sequence of information
    (2) patient categories for inpatients and outpatients

(3) indications for routine status versus STAT status

(4) color coding of different laboratories' requisitions

22. When designing a laboratory report form, which of the following factors must be included?

(1) patient identification, location, requesting M.D.

(2) date and time of specimen collection

(3) reference ranges

(4) age of the patient

23. Use of a log sheet in a specimen collection area serves what purpose(s)?

(1) keep a record of specimens collected

(2) keep confidential information available

(3) keep a record of deliveries to the laboratory

(4) keep employee salaries at hand

Answers

1. **TRUE.**

   Garza D, Becan-McBride K. Phlebotomy Handbook. E. Norwalk, CT: Appleton & Lange; 1989:169.

2. **TRUE.**

   Garza and Becan-McBride, p 171.

3. **TRUE.**

   Garza and Becan-McBride, p 174.

4. **TRUE.**

   Garza and Becan-McBride, p 190.

5. **FALSE.**

   Garza and Becan-McBride, p 183.

6. **TRUE.**

   Garza and Becan-McBride, p 183.

7. **TRUE.**

   Garza and Becan-McBride, p 182.

8. **FALSE.**

   Garza and Becan-McBride, p 182.

9. **D.**

   Garza and Becan-McBride, p 173.

10. **A.**

    Garza and Becan-McBride, p 173.

11. **B.**

    Garza and Becan-McBride, p 173.

12. **C.**

    Garza and Becan-McBride, p 173.

13. **F.**

    Garza and Becan-McBride, p 180.

14. **D.**

    Garza and Becan-McBride, p 180.

15. **E.**

    Garza and Becan-McBride, p 180.

16. **B.**

    Garza and Becan-McBride, p 180.

17. **C.**

    Garza and Becan-McBride, p 180.

18. **A.**

    Garza and Becan-McBride, p 180.

19. **A.**

    Garza and Becan-McBride, p 174.

20. **E.**

    Garza and Becan-McBride, p 179.

21. **E.**

    Garza and Becan-McBride, p 181.

22. **A.**

    Garza and Becan-McBride, p 191.

23. **B.**

    Garza and Becan-McBride, p 183.

CHAPTER 8

Interpersonal Communication Skills, Professionalism, and Liability

Questions

DIRECTIONS: Indicate whether each statement is TRUE or FALSE.

1. **True/False:** Bedside manner refers to the phlebotomist's body position while performing a venipuncture on a bedridden patient.
2. **True/False:** Most patients admit that the thing they hate most about being in the hospital is being "stuck".
3. **True/False:** A phlebotomist should never introduce himself or herself to the patient.
4. **True/False:** Patients can feel ill or faint during a glucose tolerance test.
5. **True/False:** Technical jargon should be used to explain a collection procedure to patients.
6. **True/False:** Confidentiality of patient's medical condition must be maintained by all health care workers.

DIRECTIONS: Each group of lettered words or phrases below is followed by a list of numbered words or phrases. MATCH the lettered word or phrase most closely associated with the numbered word or phrase.

Questions 7 through 11

A. Glucose tolerance test
B. Ova and parasites
C. TDM
D. 24-hour urine samples
E. Scotch tape method

7. Therapeutic drug monitoring
8. Blood and urine are taken at 30 minutes and 2, 3, 4, or 5 hours
9. Used to diagnose pinworms
10. Evaluated from stool specimens
11. Samples are collected in one container

Questions 12 through 16

A. Patient's bill of rights
B. Abraham Maslow
C. Ethics
D. Hippocratic oath
E. Florence Nightingale

12. Historical figure who affected ethical behavior for nonphysician members of the health care team
13. Describes the rights of patients in a health care environment
14. Historical pledge of behavior for physicians
15. Described theories related to human motivation
16. Principles of right and wrong

Questions 17 through 21

A. CAP
B. JCAHO
C. NPA
D. ASMT
E. ASCP

17. National Phlebotomy Association
18. College of American Pathologists
19. Joint Commission on the Accreditation of Health Care Organization
20. American Society for Medical Technology
21. American Society for Clinical Pathology

DIRECTIONS: For each of the questions or incomplete statements below, ONE or MORE of the numbered responses are correct. In each case select

A. if only 1, 2, and 3 are correct
B. if only 1 and 3 are correct
C. if only 2 and 4 are correct
D. if only 4 is correct
E. if all are correct

22. Directions to a patient for the proper collection of a 24-hour urine sample include

(1) add water to the preservative in the container
(2) void and discard urine, note the time
(3) save all urine voided for 36 hours then discard half of it
(4) save all urine voided for 24 hours

23. Good listening skills are important to a successful phlebotomist to pick up clues from a patient. To encourage a patient to expand his or her thoughts or fears, a phlebotomist might use which of the listed phrases?

(1) "Can we continue this discussion when I am off duty?"
(2) "Tell me more about it."

(3) "Are you afraid of me?"

(4) "Really?"

24. Which of the listed response phrases indicate to a patient that his or her phlebotomist is an active listener?

    (1) "Oh, I see . . ."
    (2) "Very interesting . . ."
    (3) "How about that . . ."
    (4) "When did you say it happened?"

25. Stress usually is defined by physiologic changes, such as

    (1) increased blood pressure
    (2) increased heart rate and breathing rate
    (3) increased body metabolism
    (4) increased crying

26. Imagine that a phlebotomist must collect a blood specimen from a hospitalized patient named Janie Doe. Choose the most appropriate way(s) to identify her.

    (1) ask: "Are you Ms. Janie Doe?"
    (2) ask: "What is your name?"
    (3) ask: "What is your identification number?"
    (4) check her hospital armband

27. Which of the following procedures require exact timing for specimen collection?

    (1) glucose tolerance test
    (2) therapeutic drug monitoring
    (3) 24-hour urine sample
    (4) bleeding times

28. The phlebotomist plays a very active role in patient education for which of the listed procedures?

    (1) glucose tolerance test
    (2) urine culture
    (3) 24-hour urine samples
    (4) coagulation tests

DIRECTIONS: Each of the questions or incomplete statements below is followed by suggested answers or completions. Select the BEST answer in each case.

29. A phlebotomist can make an impression on a patient within

    (A) 30 seconds
    (B) 60 seconds
    (C) 5 minutes
    (D) 1 day

30. If a patient questions the phlebotomist about what tests are ordered, what should the phlebotomist do?

    (A) indicate to the patient that the information is confidential
    (B) name the tests and refer the patient to his or her M.D.
    (C) refuse to talk
    (D) show the patient his or her medical record

DIRECTIONS: For the behaviors listed below, indicate a YES if it represents positive body language to a patient. Indicate NO if it does not represent positive body language.

31. **Yes/No:** Smiling to the patient
32. **Yes/No:** Talking to a patient at eye level
33. **Yes/No:** Resting on a patient's bed
34. **Yes/No:** Neatly groomed hair
35. **Yes/No:** Avoiding eye contact
36. **Yes/No:** Good posture
37. **Yes/No:** Standing too close to the patient
38. **Yes/No:** Rolling eyes at the ceiling
39. **Yes/No:** Yawning, stretching
40. **Yes/No:** Erect posture
41. **Yes/No:** A clean, pressed lab coat
42. **Yes/No:** A wrinkled, concerned forehead
43. **Yes/No:** Sighing, taking a deep breath

Answers

1. **FALSE.**
   Garza D, Becan-McBride K. Phlebotomy Handbook. E. Norwalk, CT: Appleton & Lange; 1989:195.

2. **TRUE.**
   Garza and Becan-McBride, p 195.

3. **FALSE.**
   Garza and Becan-McBride, p 195.

4. **TRUE.**

    Garza and Becan-McBride, p 198.

5. **FALSE.**

    Garza and Becan-McBride, p 198.

6. **TRUE.**

    Garza and Becan-McBride, p 219.

7. **C.**

    Garza and Becan-McBride, p 198.

8. **A.**

    Garza and Becan-McBride, p 198.

9. **E.**

    Garza and Becan-McBride, p 198.

10. **B.**

    Garza and Becan-McBride, p 198.

11. **D.**

    Garza and Becan-McBride, p 198.

12. **E.**

    Garza and Becan-McBride, pp 211–213.

13. **A.**

    Garza and Becan-McBride, pp 211–213.

14. **D.**

    Garza and Becan-McBride, pp 211–213.

15. **B.**

    Garza and Becan-McBride, pp 211–213.

16. **C.**

    Garza and Becan-McBride, pp 211–213.

17. **C.**

    Garza and Becan-McBride, p 224.

18. **A.**

19. **B.**

20. **D.**

    Garza and Becan-McBride, p 224.

21. **E.**

22. **C.**

    Garza and Becan-McBride, p 230–233.

23. **C.**

    Garza and Becan-McBride, p 203.

24. **A.**

    Garza and Becan-McBride, pp 202–203.

25. **C.**

    Garza and Becan-McBride, p 225.

26. **C.**

    Garza and Becan-McBride, p 196.

27. **E.**

    Garza and Becan-McBride, p 197.

28. **A.**

    Garza and Becan-McBride, p 198.

29. **A.**

    Garza and Becan-McBride, p 195.

30. **B.**

    Garza and Becan-McBride, p 195.

31. **Yes**

    Garza and Becan-McBride pp. 201–202

32. **Yes**

    Garza and Becan-McBride p. 202

33. **No**

    Garza and Becan-McBride pp. 201–202

34. **Yes**

    Garza and Becan-McBride p. 202

35. **No**

    Garza and Becan-McBride p. 202

36. **Yes**

    Garza and Becan-McBride p. 202

37. **No**

    Garza and Becan-McBride p. 202

38. **No**

    Garza and Becan-McBride pp. 201–202

39. **No**

    Garza and Becan-McBride pp. 201–202

40. **Yes**

    Garza and Becan-McBride pp. 201–202

41. **Yes**

    Garza and Becan-McBride pp. 201–202

42. **No**

    Garza and Becan-McBride p. 202

43. **No**

    Garza and Becan-McBride p. 202

CHAPTER 9

Quality Assurance and Safety in Blood Collection

Questions

DIRECTIONS: Each of the questions or incomplete statements below is followed by suggested answers or completions. Select the BEST answer in each case.

1. The monitoring or assuring of all procedures from the time the patient's blood specimen is obtained until the time laboratory results are reported is called

   (A) disinfection assurance
   (B) quality control
   (C) quality assurance
   (D) infection control

2. The first step in controlling severe bleeding is to

   (A) send for medical assistance
   (B) start cardiopulmonary resuscitation
   (C) apply pressure directly over the wound or venipuncture site
   (D) make the individual lie down and apply pressure on the person's forehead

3. Although aseptic technique is important in all blood collection procedures, it is of the utmost importance in the collection of which of the following specimens?

   (A) blood gases
   (B) crossmatch
   (C) blood culture
   (D) creatinine

4. Which of the following organizations provides accreditation to those clinical laboratories that maintain a proper quality assurance plan and program?

   (A) College of American Pathologist
   (B) College of American Laboratories
   (C) College of American Phlebotomists
   (D) Joint Commission of Laboratory Scientists

5. Which of the following terms implies operational procedures used to implement the quality assurance program?

   (A) quality assurance
   (B) quality control
   (C) infection control
   (D) infection assurance

6. As a rule of thumb, the volume of blood drawn should be equal to _____ times the amount of serum or plasma required for a laboratory assay?

   (A) 1½
   (B) 2½
   (C) 3½
   (D) 5½

DIRECTIONS: For each of the questions or incomplete statements below, ONE or MORE of the numbered responses are correct. In each case select

   A. if only 1, 2, and 3 are correct
   B. if only 1 and 3 are correct
   C. if only 2 and 4 are correct
   D. if only 4 is correct
   E. if all are correct

7. Which of the following is/are examples of physiologic conditions that the phlebotomist should be aware of for quality assurance in specimen collection?

   (1) the effects of changes in the patient's posture
   (2) the effects of diurnal variation
   (3) the effects of the patient exercising
   (4) the effects of the patient's diet for 3 days preceding the glucose tolerance test

8. Which of the following may cause inaccurate laboratory test results?

   (1) nonfasting patient
   (2) misidentified or mislabeled specimen

(3) repeated freezing and thawing of a specimen

(4) collecting a blood specimen from a patient who won a marathon the preceding day

9. Which of the following should be considered when choosing a specimen transport container?

(1) cost

(2) temperature control needs

(3) sturdiness and durability

(4) type of label

10. If a patient is having a fasting laboratory test performed and the patient did not fast, the phlebotomist should note this problem on the

(1) physician's notes

(2) medical technologist's notes

(3) patient's medical chart

(4) patient's laboratory requisition

11. Which of the following organizations provide accreditation to those clinical laboratories that maintain a proper quality assurance plan and program?

(1) American Association of Bioanalysts

(2) Joint Commission of Pathologists

(3) College of American Pathologists

(4) American Association of Phlebotomists

12. Which of the following is/are steps included in a quality assurance program?

(1) identification of potential problems

(2) establishment of priorities to confront the problem

(3) provision of procedures to monitor continually the activities that have been established to correct the problem

(4) documentation to demonstrate that the quality assurance plan is effective and efficient in providing quality patient care

DIRECTIONS: Indicate whether each statement is TRUE or FALSE.

13. **True/False:** Table 9–1 is an example of a page from a floor book that describes preparation of the patient and special handling of patients' specimens.

TABLE 9–1.

Test	Sample Fluid	Sample Minimum Volume (mL)	Special Handling	Reference Range	Days Available	Usual Reporting Time
Blood gases	WB (heparin)	1	Arterial blood collected in a heparinized syringe; transport on ice	pH 7.35–7.45 Po_2 88–108 mm Hg Pco_2 35–45 mm Hg	All (all)	10 min
Bromide	S	4		Th 1–2 mg/mL	M–F (9AM)	8 hr
Bromsulphalein clearance	S	3	Collect 45 min after administration of dye	< 7% retention	M–F (9 AM)	8 hr
Calcium, ionized	S	2	Collect on ice; submit immediately	2.20–2.60 mEq/L	M–F (9 AM)	8 hr
Calcium total	S	2		8.5–10.5 mg/dL	All (all)	8 hr
	U	10	24-hr timed specimen Add 10 mL conc. HCl to bottle prior to collection	40–220 mg/24 hr	All (9 AM)	8 hr
Carbamazepine	S	1		Th 2–12 µg/mL	M–F (9 AM, 5 PM)	8 hr
	S	2		24–32 mEq/L	All (all)	4 hr
Carbon dioxide content	U	0.5	CALL PATHOLOGIST			

14. **True/False:** For an infant weighing from 6 to 8 pounds, the maximum amount of blood to be drawn at any one time is 30 mL.

15. **True/False:** For a patient under 14 years old and weighing 96 to 100 pounds, the maximum amount of blood to be drawn at any one time is 30 mL.

16. **True/False:** The components of fire are fuel and heat plus the necessary chain reaction.

17. **True/False:** The cardinal principles in protecting oneself from radiation exposure are time, shielding, and distance.

18. **True/False:** Figure 9–1 is a sign for possible biohazardous materials.

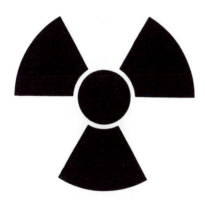

Figure 9–1.

19. **True/False:** When breathing movements stop or lips, tongue, and fingernails become blue, immediate mouth-to-mouth resuscitation is needed.

20. **True/False:** To prevent shock, it is important to give fluids to an unconscious or semiconscious person.

DIRECTIONS: Each group of lettered words or phrases below is followed by a list of numbered words or phrases. MATCH the lettered word or phrase most closely associated with the numbered word or phrase.

Questions 21 through 25

A. breathing aid
B. chemical spill
C. stopping bleeding
D. circulation aid
E. preventing shock

21. CPR
22. Improve circulation, provide sufficient oxygen, and maintain normal body temperature
23. Quickly give four ventilations
24. A clean handkerchief or other clean cloth should be used and then pressure applied
25. A clean-up kit with absorbents and neutralizers should be obtained

Questions 26 through 30

A. fire safety
B. electrical safety
C. radiation safety
D. chemical safety
E. mechanical safety

26. If the carriers are not in the correct position, they can swing out of the holding discs
27. Carefully read the label before using any reagent
28. Asbestos gloves or a glass beaker should be used in this type of accident to provide safety to the rescuer
29. Four general classifications have been adopted and four extinguishers correspond
30. Time, shielding, and distance are the principles of protection

DIRECTIONS: For each of the questions or incomplete statements below, ONE or MORE of the numbered responses are correct. In each case select

A. if only 1, 2, and 3 are correct
B. if only 1 and 3 are correct
C. if only 2 and 4 are correct
D. if only 4 is correct
E. if all are correct

31. If a fire occurs in or near electrical equipment, which of the following fire extinguishers should be used?

(1) ABC extinguisher
(2) class A extinguisher
(3) class C extinguisher
(4) class B extinguisher

32. A fasting blood specimen is needed for which of the following clinical laboratory assays?

(1) triglycerides
(2) glucose
(3) cholesterol
(4) hematocrit

33. Which of the listed operational procedures should be followed for quality control on evacuated blood collection tubes?

(1) check for clots by straining anticoagulated blood through gauze
(2) sample spin down
(3) check for vacuum draw
(4) visual inspection for anticoagulants

34. A fasting blood specimen for glucose analysis is collected in the morning rather than at a random collection time for which of the following reasons?

    (1) to enhance the effects of diurnal variation
    (2) to avoid the effects of food intake
    (3) to avoid the effects of exercise
    (4) to enhance the phlebotomist's schedule

35. Which of the following laboratory assays could have a designated delivery time of 20 minutes without harm to the outcome of the laboratory results?

    (1) electrolytes
    (2) enzymes
    (3) chemistry profile
    (4) feces for ameba identification

36. Which of the following items is/are usually included in a laboratory written procedure on the inability to draw specimens?

    (1) unsuccessful collection attempts
    (2) patient unavailability
    (3) patient refusal
    (4) phlebotomist unavailability

37. Which of the following statements is/are true concerning Figure 9–2?

    (1) on day 10, the glucose control had a mean value of 100 mg/dL
    (2) on day 8, the glucose control was out of the ± 2 standard deviation level
    (3) on day 2, the glucose control read 103 mg/dL
    (4) on day 5, the glucose control was the same as the patient's glucose value

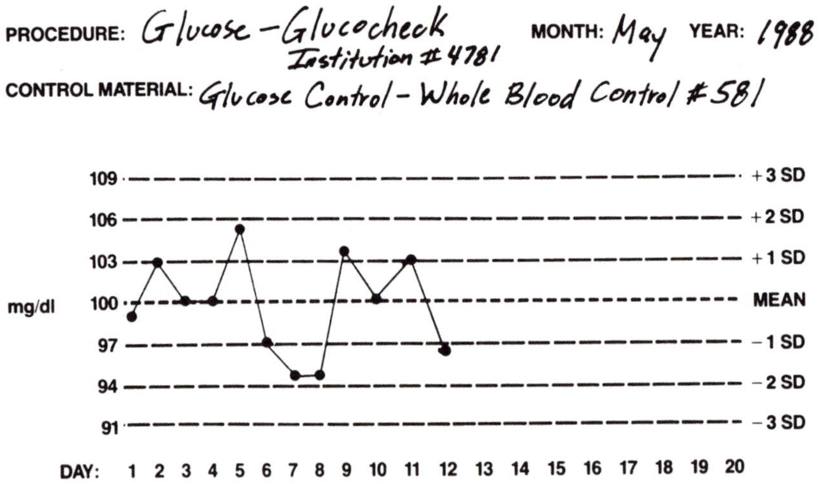

PROCEDURE: *Glucose –Glucocheck* MONTH: *May* YEAR: *1988*
  Institution #4781

CONTROL MATERIAL: *Glucose Control – Whole Blood Control #581*

Figure 9–2. *Clinical chemistry quality control chart. From Garza, D., and Becan-McBride, K.* Phlebotomy Handbook, second edition. *Norwalk, Ct: Appleton & Lange; 1989.*

38. In Table 9–2A, insert the following designated delivery times for the appropriate laboratory assays.
    Designated delivery times:
    Immediately
    20 minutes
    90 minutes

TABLE 9–2A. EXAMPLES OF DESIGNATED DELIVERY TIMES FOR LABORATORY SPECIMENS

Clinical Microbiology	
Routine bacterial culture	
Swab with holding medium	_____
Swab without holding medium	_____
Body fluids	40 min
Parasitology	
Feces for ameba identification	_____
Clinical Chemistry	
Glucose	_____
Enzymes	30 min
Chemical profile	30 min
Urinalysis/Clinical Microscopy	
Routine urinalysis	_____

DIRECTIONS: Indicate whether each statement is TRUE or FALSE.

39. True/False: In case of a chemical spill in the eye, the victim should rinse his or her eyes at the eyewash station for a minimum of 15 minutes before removing his or her contact lenses.

40. True/False: If first aid is given to a shock victim and the victim appears to have no broken bones, elevate the victim's legs so that the head is lower than the trunk of the body.

41. True/False: If a fire occurs with ordinary combustible materials, such as wood, rubbish, and paper, class A extinguishers should be used to cool the fire and put it out.

42. True/False: To determine the rate and possible source of blood culture contamination, the clinical microbiology section of the laboratory may maintain a written or computer log to tabulate negative and positive results and contaminated specimens.

43. True/False: As shown in Figure 9–3, a collection log on pediatric and newborn patients should be maintained to keep the phlebotomist busy when he or she has no blood collection activities.

Week __1__   Month __March__   Year __1988__
Collection Log on Pediatric and Newborn Patients

Date	Patient	Age	Patient Number	Floor	Test Requested	Amount Collected
3-4-84	Rubinoff, Baby	4 days	1650421	NB Nur	SMAC 20	3 microtainers
3-4-84	Gustafson, H.	5 yrs	177482	6B	electrolytes	$2 \times 250\ \mu l$
3-4-84	Benson, J.	12 mo	185621	6B	Hb & Hct	$2 \times 20\ \mu l$

Figure 9–3. Blood collections on pediatric and newborn patients. *(Courtesy of Hermann Hospital Clinical Laboratory, Houston, TX.)*

DIRECTIONS: Each group of lettered words or phrases below is followed by a list of numbered words or phrases. MATCH the lettered word or phrase most closely associated with the numbered word or phrase.

Questions 44 through 48

A. the patient must ingest at least 300 g of carbohydrates daily for at least 3 days before this test

44. Total serum calcium
45. Urinary total catecholamines

B. 10 mL of concentrated HCl is added to bottle before collection
C. one clotted blood specimen is required
D. collect and transport on ice; submit immediately
E. arterial blood collected in a heparinized syringe; transport on ice

46. GTT
47. Blood gases
48. Ionized calcium

Questions 49 through 53

A. National Committee for Clinical Laboratory Standards
B. College of American Pathologists
C. Centers for Disease Control
D. QCPM
E. NBS

49. Provides accreditation to those clinical laboratories that maintain a proper quality assurance plan and program
50. Quality control and preventive maintenance
51. The anticoagulants and preservatives used in blood collection should meet the requirements of this organization
52. National Bureau of Standards
53. Provides regulations regarding shipment of biologic specimens

DIRECTIONS: For each of the questions or incomplete statements below, ONE or MORE of the numbered responses are correct. In each case select

A. if only 1, 2, and 3 are correct
B. if only 1 and 3 are correct
C. if only 2 and 4 are correct
D. if only 4 is correct
E. if all are correct

54. Which of the following applies/apply to the transportation of blood specimens through the United States Postal Service (USPS)? The USPS

(1) bans all blood specimens from being transported through the USPS mail
(2) does not accept blood specimens for USPS mail unless the clinical specimens are intended for "medical or veterinary use, research, or laboratory certification related to public health"
(3) does not accept blood specimens for USPS mail unless it is an emergency situation

tainer system with the outer shipping container labeled to indicate "Etiologic Agents/Biohazard Material"

55. Which of the following statement(s) is/are true for maintenance and
quality control procedures regarding the centrifuge?

(1) the speed of the centrifuge can be checked by a tachometer
(2) the speed of the centrifuge is indicated by the unit mm Hg
(3) the g value for the centrifuge gives the efficiency of the instrument
(4) the relative centrifugal force is the same as revolutions per minute

56. Which of the following instrument(s) is/are used in bedside glucose
testing?

(1) Accu-Check II
(2) Glucocheck
(3) Diascan
(4) Glucometer II

57. Which of the following statements is/are true for maintenance and
quality control procedures regarding the sphygmomanometer?

(1) the unit of measurement on the sphygmomanometer dial is
mm Hg
(2) the gauge of the sphygmomanometer should be tested against a
calibrated sphygmomanometer gauge for accuracy
(3) accuracy checks on sphygmomanometers should be performed
at least on a quarterly basis
(4) a difference of more than 25 mm Hg in the reading of the
tested sphygmomanometer versus the calibrated sphygmomanometer is acceptable

58. Which of the following statements lead(s) to safety in specimen collection?

(1) it is okay to apply cosmetics on the job if the phlebotomist
washes her hands first
(2) eating within the specimen control section and other laboratory
sections must be avoided
(3) as long as the laboratory coat is worn completely buttoned
while collecting specimens, it is okay to wear it during lunch
and coffee breaks
(4) the phlebotomist should avoid biting her or his fingernails or
rubbing the eyes

DIRECTIONS: Each of the questions or incomplete statements below is followed by suggested answers or completions. Select the BEST answer in each case.

59. Safe working conditions must be ensured by the employer and have been mandated by law under the

    (A) Occupational Safety and Health Act
    (B) Institutional Safety and Health Act
    (C) Health Care Facility Institutional Safety Act
    (D) Health Care Facility and Occupational Safety Act

60. If an accident occurs, such as sticking oneself with a needle after performing venipuncture on a patient, the first thing that the phlebotomist should do is

    (A) contact her or his immediate supervisor
    (B) fill out the necessary health care forms
    (C) cleanse the area with isopropyl alcohol and apply a Band-Aid
    (D) take the needle back to the clinical laboratory for verification of the accident

61. If a phlebotomist is in an area of the health care facility where a fire starts, she or he should do which of the following first?

    (A) attempt to extinguish the fire, using the proper extinguisher
    (B) pull the fire alarm box
    (C) close all doors and windows before leaving the area
    (D) block the entrances so that others will not enter the fire area

62. The phlebotomist is most likely to encounter which of the following hazards on entering the nuclear medicine department to obtain a blood specimen from a patient?

    (A) fire hazard
    (B) radiation hazard
    (C) mechanical hazard
    (D) electrical hazard

63. NBS is an abbreviation for

    (A) National Board Standard
    (B) National Board Statistics
    (C) National Bureau of Statistics
    (D) National Bureau of Standards

64. In terms of quality control procedures, SD stands for

    (A) short distance
    (B) standard deviation
    (C) shared diameter
    (D) standard dimension

65. On a quality control chart, interpretation of the chart is based on the fact that for a normal distribution

    (A) 99% of the values are within ± 3 SD of the mean
    (B) 99% of the values are within ± 2 SD of the mean
    (C) 95% of the values are within ± 3 SD of the mean
    (D) 95% of the values are within ± 1 SD of the mean

DIRECTIONS: Indicate whether each statement is TRUE or FALSE.

66. **True/False:** When transporting acids or alkalis, an acid carrier should be used.
67. **True/False:** In the clinical laboratory, it is quite appropriate to dispose of used blood specimen equipment in any waste container that has a lid.
68. **True/False:** As shown in Figure 9–2 (page 146), the glucose control– whole blood control No. 581 has a mean value of 100 mg/dL on days 3, 4, and 10.
69. **True/False:** In a health care institution, if a patient refuses to have his or her blood drawn, the phlebotomist should demand the patient's cooperation in order to obtain the needed blood specimen(s).
70. **True/False:** To calibrate a thermometer, the thermometer should be tested against an NBS-certified thermometer within or near the temperature ranges intended for use.
71. **True/False:** In the performance of bedside glucose testing, a fingerstick usually is performed, and the first drop of blood is applied by allowing the drop to fall from the finger onto the strip or reagent pad.

DIRECTIONS: Each group of lettered words or phrases below is followed by a list of numbered words or phrases. MATCH the lettered word or phrase most closely associated with the numbered word or phrase.

Questions 72 through 76

A. ± 2 SD from the mean   72. RCF
B. mm Hg   73. Units for blood glucose

C. *g* value
D. mg/dL
E. ± 3 SD from the mean

74. 99% of the values about the average
75. 95% of the values about the average
76. Units on a sphygmomanometer

Questions 77 through 81

A. rpm
B. minimum index (L) and maximum index (H)
C. aneroid gauge should be within 0 reading
D. uses reagent strips
E. contains foam, dry chemical, or carbon dioxide

77. Sphygmomanometer
78. Centrifuge
79. Class B extinguisher
80. Thermometer
81. Glucometer II

DIRECTIONS: Each of the questions or incomplete statements below is followed by suggested answers or completions. Select the BEST answer in each case.

82. If a phlebotomist is caught in a fire in the health care institution, he or she should not do which of the following?

    (A) run
    (B) close all doors and windows before leaving the area
    (C) if the fire is small, attempt to extinguish it, using the proper equipment
    (D) call the assigned fire number

83. For safety in the clinical laboratory, which of the following should not occur?

    (A) needles, syringes, and lancets should be disposed of in a special sturdy container
    (B) liquid waste should be discarded rapidly to be rid of it quickly
    (C) specimen control section should be disinfected periodically according to the clinical laboratory schedule
    (D) patients' specimens should be covered at all times during transportation

84. Which of the following actions is not part of the quality control (QC) activities to take place when a new lot number of evacuated blood collection tubes is placed into use? The new lot number of tubes should be checked for

    (A) metals contamination
    (B) glucose content

(C) sterility of tube (if indicated)

(D) clots by straining anticoagulated blood through gauge

85. Which of the following instruments usually is not found in the specimen control area of the laboratory?

(A) thermometer

(B) centrifuge

(C) sphygmomanometer

(D) fluorometer

Answers and Explanations

1. **C.** Quality assurance is the monitoring or assuring of all procedures from the time a patient's blood specimen is obtained until the time laboratory results are reported.
   Garza D, Becan-McBride K. Phlebotomy Handbook. *E. Norwalk, CT: Appleton & Lange; 1989:229.*

2. **C.** The first step in controlling severe bleeding is to apply pressure directly over the wound or venipuncture site.
   Garza and Becan-McBride, p 252.

3. **C.** Aseptic technique is of the utmost importance in the collection of a blood culture specimen from a patient.
   Garza and Becan-McBride, p 241.

4. **A.** The College of American Pathologists (CAP) provides accreditation to those clinical laboratories that maintain a proper quality assurance plan and program.
   Garza and Becan-McBride, p 229.

5. **B.** Quality control implies operational procedures used to implement the quality assurance program.
   Garza and Becan-McBride, p 230.

6. **B.** As a rule of thumb, the volume of blood drawn should equal 2½ times the amount of serum or plasma required.
   Garza and Becan-McBride, p 235.

7. **E.** Examples of patient preparation necessary for quality assurance in specimen collection include the effects of (1) changes in the patient's posture, (2) diurnal variation, (3) the patient exercising, and (4) the patient's diet for 3 days before the glucose tolerance test.
   Garza and Becan-McBride, p 233.

8. **E.** Inaccurate laboratory test results may be caused by (1) collecting blood from a nonfasting patient when a fasting specimen is necessary,

(2) a misidentified or mislabeled specimen, (3) repeated freezing and thawing of a specimen, and (4) collecting a blood specimen from a patient who has been exercising vigorously on the day before the laboratory testing.

Garza and Becan-McBride, pp 233, 237–238.

9. **E.** When choosing a specimen transport container, the following issues should be considered: (1) cost, (2) temperature control needs of the specimen, (3) sturdiness and durability, and (4) type of label (e.g., cloth, special plastic).

Garza and Becan-McBride, pp 235–237.

10. **D.** If a patient is having a fasting laboratory test performed and the patient did not fast, the phlebotomist should note this on the patient's laboratory requisition.

Garza and Becan-McBride, pp 238–239.

11. **B.** The American Association of Bioanalysts and the College of American Pathologists are two organizations that provide accreditation to those clinical laboratories that maintain a proper quality assurance plan and program.

Garza and Becan-McBride, p 229.

12. **E.** The steps included in a quality assurance program are (1) identification of potential problems in such a program, (2) provision of objective evaluation of the cause and extent of the problem, (3) establishment of priorities to confront the problem, (4) provision of activities to correct the problem, (5) provision of procedures to continually monitor the activities that have been established to correct the problem, and (6) documentation to demonstrate that the quality assurance plan is effective and efficient in providing quality patient care.

Garza and Becan-McBride, pp 229–230.

13. **TRUE.** Table 9–1 is an example of a page from a floor book that describes preparation of the patient and special handling of patient's specimens.

Garza and Becan-McBride, p 231.

14. **FALSE.** For an infant weighing 6 to 8 pounds, the maximum amount of blood to be drawn at any one time is 2.5 mL.

Garza and Becan-McBride, p 241.

15. **TRUE.** For a patient under 14 years old and weighing 96 to 100 pounds, the maximum amount of blood to be drawn at any one time is 30 mL.

Garza and Becan-McBride, p 241.

16. **FALSE.** The components of fire are fuel, oxygen, and heat, plus the necessary chain reaction.

Garza and Becan-McBride, p 248.

17. **TRUE.** The cardinal principles in protecting oneself from radiation exposure are time, shielding, and distance.
    Garza and Becan-McBride, p 249.

18. **FALSE.** Figure 9–1 is a sign for possible radiation hazard.
    Garza and Becan-McBride, p 250.

19. **TRUE.** When breathing movements stop or lips, tongue, and fingernails become blue, immediate mouth-to-mouth resuscitation is needed.
    Garza and Becan-McBride, p 252.

20. **FALSE.** It is extremely important not to give fluids to an unconscious or semiconscious person.
    Garza and Becan-McBride, p 254.

21. **D.** In order to maintain circulation in a patient or other victim, the phlebotomist must know the techniques of basic cardiopulmonary resuscitation (CPR).
    Garza and Becan-McBride, p 254.

22. **E.** The main objectives in treating a shock victim are to improve circulation, provide sufficient oxygen, and maintain normal body temperature.
    Garza and Becan-McBride, p 254.

23. **A.** As shown in Figure 9–4, if a victim is not breathing, the victim's head should be tilted after checking for obstructions in the mouth or throat. Then pinch the victim's nose shut, open mouth wide, take a deep breath, and quickly give four ventilations.
    Garza and Becan-McBride, p 252.

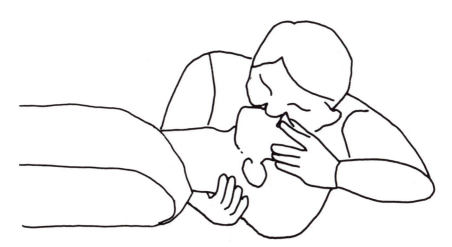

Figure 9—4. Breathing aid in emergency situation. *(Adapted from the American Heart Assocation, with permission.)*

24. **C.** A clean handkerchief or other clean cloth (compress) should be placed over the wound before applying pressure by the hand.
Garza and Becan-McBride, p 252.

25. **B.** If a chemical spill occurs, the phlebotomist should obtain a spill clean-up kit from the clinical chemistry section. The kit includes absorbents and neutralizers.
Garza and Becan-McBride, p 251.

26. **E.** If the carriers of the centrifuge are not in the correct position, they can swing out of the holding discs into the side of the centrifuge.
Garza and Becan-McBride, p 250.

27. **D.** Because the phlebotomist must sometimes pour preservatives, such as HCl, into containers for 24-hour urine collections and transport these to the patients' floors, he or she should read the label carefully before using the reagents.
Garza and Becan-McBride, p 250.

28. **B.** If an electrical accident occurs involving electrical shock to some employee or patient, the phlebotomist should be aware of the following: (1) the electrical power source must be shut off, (2) if this is impossible, carefully remove the electrical contact from the victim using something, such as asbestos gloves, that does not conduct electricity or place one's hand in a glass beaker and push the power supply away from the victim.
Garza and Becan-McBride, p 249.

29. **A.** Four general classifications of fire have been adopted by the National Fire Protection Association, and fire extinguishers correspond with each class of fire.
Garza and Becan-McBride, p 248.

30. **C.** The three cardinal principles in protecting oneself from radiation exposure are time, shielding, and distance.
Garza and Becan-McBride, p 249.

31. **B.** If a fire occurs in or near electrical equipment, a multipurpose (ABC) or class C extinguisher can be used.
Garza and Becan-McBride, p 248.

32. **A.** A fasting blood specimen is needed for the testing of triglyceride, cholesterol, and glucose levels.
Garza and Becan-McBride, p 233.

33. **E.** In order to have quality control on evacuated blood collection tubes, the following operational procedures should be followed: (1) check for clots by straining anticoagulated blood through gauze, (2)

sample spin down, (3) check for vacuum draw, and (4) conduct a visual inspection for anticoagulants.

Garza and Becan-McBride, p 234.

34. **A.** A fasting blood specimen for glucose analysis is collected in the morning rather than at a random collection time in order to (1) enhance the effects of diurnal variation, (2) avoid the effects of food intake, and (3) avoid the effects of exercise.

Garza and Becan-McBride, p 233.

35. **A.** The electrolytes (Na^+, K^+, Cl^-, HCO_3^-), enzymes, and chemistry profiles can be run on blood collected in the designated delivery time of 20 minutes.

Garza and Becan-McBride, p 238.

36. **A.** The items usually included in a laboratory written procedure on the inability to draw specimens include the steps that should be taken by the phlebotomist in (1) unsuccessful collection attempts, (2) patient unavailability, and (3) patient refusal.

Garza and Becan-McBride, p 239.

37. **B.** From reviewing Figure 9–2, it can be determined that on day 10, the glucose control had a mean value of 100 mg/dL, and on day 2, the glucose control read 103 mg/dL.

Garza and Becan-McBride, p 245.

38.

TABLE 9–2B. EXAMPLES OF DESIGNATED DELIVERY TIMES FOR LABORATORY SPECIMENS

Clinical Microbiology	
Routine bacterial culture	
Swab with holding medium	90 min
Swab without holding medium	20 min
Body fluids	40 min
Parasitology	
Feces for ameba identification	Immediately
Clinical Chemistry	
Glucose	20 min
Enzymes	30 min
Chemical profile	30 min
Urinalysis/Clinical Microscopy	
Routine urinalysis	90 min

Garza and Becan-McBride, p 238.

39. **FALSE.** In case of a chemical spill in the eye, the victim should rinse his or her eyes at the eyewash station for a minimum of 15 minutes. Contact lenses must be removed before the rinsing in order to cleanse the eyes thoroughly.
Garza and Becan-McBride, p 251.

40. **TRUE.** If first aid is given to a shock victim and the victim appears to have no broken bones, elevate the victim's legs so that the head is lower than the trunk of the body.
Garza and Becan-McBride, p 254.

41. **TRUE.** If a fire occurs with ordinary combustible materials, such as wood, rubbish, and paper, a class A extinguisher containing soda and acid or water should be used to cool the fire.
Garza and Becan-McBride, p 248.

42. **TRUE.** To determine the rate and possible source of blood culture contamination, the clinical microbiology section may maintain a written or computer log to tabulate negative and positive culture results and contaminated specimens.
Garza and Becan-McBride, p 241.

43. **FALSE.** As shown in Figure 9–3, a collection log on pediatric and newborn patients should be maintained. Because of their blood volume, it is best to collect the minimum required amount of blood for each laboratory assay to avoid significant blood loss during their hospital stay.
Garza and Becan-McBride, p 239.

44. **C.** In order to determine a total serum calcium level on a patient, a dotted blood sample is needed.
Garza and Becan-McBride, p 231.

45. **B.** Urinary total catecholamines must be collected with 10 mL of concentrated HCl.
Garza and Becan-McBride, p 232.

46. **A.** The patient must ingest at least 300 g of carbohydrates daily for at least 3 days before the glucose tolerance test (GTT).
Garza and Becan-McBride, p 233.

47. **E.** To determine levels of blood gases, arterial blood is collected in a heparinized syringe and transported on ice.
Garza and Becan-McBride, p 231.

48. **D.** To obtain a patient's ionized calcium level, collected blood must be transported on ice and submitted immediately.
Garza and Becan-McBride, p 231.

49. **B.** The College of American Pathologists (CAP) provides accreditation to those clinical laboratories that maintain a proper quality assurance plan and program.
Garza and Becan-McBride, p 229.

50. **D.** QCPM is an abbreviation for quality control and preventive maintenance.
Garza and Becan-McBride, p 242.

51. **A.** In order to assure quality, the anticoagulants and preservatives used in blood collection should meet the requirements established by the National Committee for Clinical Laboratory Standards.
Garza and Becan-McBride, pp 233–234.

52. **E.** NBS is an abbreviation for National Bureau of Standards.
Garza and Becan-McBride, p 243.

53. **C.** The Centers for Disease Control (CDC) provides regulations regarding shipment of biologic specimens.
Garza and Becan-McBride, p 237.

54. **C.** The United States Postal Service (USPS) (1) does not accept blood specimens for mail unless the clinical specimens are intended for "medical or veterinary use, research, or laboratory certification related to public health" and (2) requires that the blood specimen be transported in a dual container system with the outer shipping container labeled to indicate "Etiologic Agents/Biohazard Material."
Garza and Becan-McBride, pp 236–237; Federal Register August 15, 1989; 54(156):33523–33525.

55. **B.** The speed of the centrifuge can be checked by a tachometer that indicates the speed in revolutions per minute. The relative centrifugal force or g value for the centrifuge gives the efficiency of the instrument.
Garza and Becan-McBride, p 244.

56. **E.** Examples of bedside glucose monitoring instruments include Accu-Check II (Boehringer Mannheim Diagnostics, Indianapolis, IN), Glucocheck (Larken Industries, Ltd., Lenexa, KS), Diascan (HDI, Home Diagnostics, Inc., Eatontown, NJ), and Glucometer II (Ames Division, Miles Laboratories, Elkhart, IN).
Garza and Becan-McBride, p 245.

57. **A.** The following statements are true for the maintenance and quality control procedures regarding the sphygmomanometer: (1) the unit of measurement on the sphygmomanometer dial is mm Hg, (2) the gauge of the sphygmomanometer should be tested against a calibrated sphygmomanometer gauge for accuracy, and (3) accuracy checks on sphygmomanometers should be performed at least quarterly.
Garza and Becan-McBride, p 243.

58. **C.** The following actions lead to safety in specimen collection: (1) eating within the specimen control section and other laboratory sections must be avoided, and (2) the phlebotomist should avoid biting his or her fingernails or rubbing the eyes.

    Garza and Becan-McBride, p 246.

59. **A.** Safe working conditions must be ensured by the employer and have been mandated by law under the Occupational Safety and Health Act (OSHA).

    Garza and Becan-McBride, p 246.

60. **C.** If an accident occurs, such as sticking oneself with a needle after performing venipuncture on a patient, the phlebotomist should immediately cleanse the area with isopropyl alcohol and apply a Band-Aid.

    Garza and Becan-McBride, p 247.

61. **B.** If a phlebotomist is in an area of the health care facility where a fire starts, he or she should first pull the fire alarm box.

    Garza and Becan-McBride, p 248.

62. **B.** The phlebotomist is most likely to encounter a radiation hazard when he or she enters the nuclear medicine department to obtain a blood specimen from a patient.

    Garza and Becan-McBride, pp 249–250.

63. **D.** NBS is an abbreviation for National Bureau of Standards.

    Garza and Becan-McBride, p 243.

64. **B.** In terms of quality control procedures, SD stands for standard deviation.

    Garza and Becan-McBride, p 246.

65. **A.** On a quality control chart, the interpretation of the chart is based on the fact that for a normal distribution, 99% of the values are within ± 3 SD of the mean.

    Garza and Becan-McBride, p 246.

66. **TRUE.** For chemical safety, when transporting acids or alkalis, an acid carrier should be used.

    Garza and Becan-McBride, pp 250–251.

67. **FALSE.** All waste from specimen collection must be disposed of in the correct containers. One container is usually a heavy double plastic bag that is used for disposal of blood specimens. There is another container for gauze and general trash, and a special container for needles, syringes, and lancets.

    Garza and Becan-McBride, p 247.

68. **TRUE.** As shown in Figure 9–2, the glucose control–whole blood control No. 581 has a mean value of 100 mg/dL on days 3, 4, and 10.
Garza and Becan-McBride, p 245.

69. **FALSE.** If a patient refuses to have his or her blood drawn, the phlebotomist should notify the primary nurse and leave the requisition slips at the unit desk with the following information: (1) patient refused, (2) time and initials of phlebotomist, and (3) name of nurse notified.
Garza and Becan-McBride, p 240.

70. **TRUE.** To calibrate a thermometer, the thermometer should be tested against an NBS-certified thermometer within or near the temperature ranges intended for use.
Garza and Becan-McBride, p 242.

71. **FALSE.** In the performance of bedside glucose testing, a fingerstick usually is performed. The first drop of blood is wiped away, and the next drop is applied by allowing the drop to fall from the finger onto the strip or reagent pad.
Garza and Becan-McBride, 245.

72. **C.** The relative centrifugal force (RCF) also is referred to as the g value.
Garza and Becan-McBride, p 244.

73. **D.** The blood glucose values are reported in mg/dL units.
Garza and Becan-McBride, p 245.

74. **E.** For interpretation of the quality control chart, 99% of the values are between ± 3 SD from the average (mean).
Garza and Becan-McBride, p 246.

75. **A.** For interpretation of the quality control chart, 95% of the values are between ± 2 SD from the average (mean).
Garza and Becan-McBride, p 246.

76. **B.** Sphygmomanometers have a gauge with mm Hg.
Garza and Becan-McBride, p 243.

77. **C.** The sphygmomanometer has an aneroid gauge that should be within the 0 reading.
Garza and Becan-McBride, p 243.

78. **A.** The speed of a centrifuge can be checked by a tachometer that indicates the speed in revolutions per minute (rpm).
Garza and Becan-McBride, p 244.

79. **E.** Class B extinguishers contain foam, dry chemical, or carbon dioxide to combat fires composed of vapor–air mixtures over solvents.
    Garza and Becan-McBride, p 248.

80. **B.** For quality control preventive maintenance (QCPM) procedures on a Taylor Maximum–Minimum thermometer, the minimum index (L) and maximum index (H) must be recorded on a daily basis.
    Garza and Becan-McBride, p 243.

81. **D.** The Glucometer II (Ames Division, Miles Laboratories, Elkhart, IN) uses reagent strips to determine blood glucose levels.
    Garza and Becan-McBride, p 245.

82. **A.** If a phlebotomist is caught in a fire in the health care institution, he or she should not run.
    Garza and Becan-McBride, p 249.

83. **B.** Liquid waste must be disposed of gently so that liquids do not splash on other objects.
    Garza and Becan-McBride, p 247.

84. **B.** Checking for glucose content is not part of the quality control activities to take place when a new lot number of evacuated blood collection tubes is placed into use.
    Garza and Becan-McBride, p 234.

85. **D.** The fluorometer usually is not found in the specimen control area of the laboratory.
    Garza and Becan-McBride, pp 242–246.

CHAPTER 10

Management and Education

Questions

DIRECTIONS: Each of the questions or incomplete statements below is followed by suggested answers or completions. Select the BEST answer in each case.

1. To plan the implementation of a phlebotomy unit, which of the following must be considered first?

   (A) the space and facilities that will be available for the phlebotomy unit
   (B) the goals and mission of the hospital, agency, clinic, or company
   (C) the number of phlebotomists to be hired as employees
   (D) the phlebotomy supplies and equipment that must be ordered for the phlebotomy unit to function

2. Which of the following should indicate to a great extent the types of supplies and equipment that are needed in a phlebotomy unit?

   (A) the nurse administrator's desires
   (B) the medical specialties of the physicians in the health care institution (e.g., pediatrics, oncology, geriatrics)
   (C) the physical therapy specialties within the health care institution
   (D) the type of x-ray equipment that is located near the clinical laboratory

3. For budgeting in the phlebotomy section of the clinical laboratory, which of the following budgets is typically used?

   (A) outlook budget
   (B) zero base budget

(C) base 10 budget
(D) forecast budget

4. Which of the following provides an example of fixed cost in a budget?

(A) phlebotomy supplies
(B) evacuated blood collection tubes
(C) space, utilities, administration
(D) microtainers, tourniquets, disposable gloves

5. Which major management activity dictates the importance of overseeing the other management activities and leads to necessary adjustments?

(A) planning
(B) monitoring
(C) organizing
(D) criticizing

6. It is generally agreed that the best leadership approach is

(A) authoritarian
(B) dictatorship
(C) participative type
(D) autocratic type

7. In phlebotomy management, the term FTE stands for

(A) factor time equivalent
(B) full-time equation
(C) factor-temperature equation
(D) full-time employee

8. The most important resource in accomplishing the objectives of the phlebotomy unit are the

(A) inpatients
(B) outpatients
(C) phlebotomists
(D) hospital administrators

DIRECTIONS: Each group of lettered words or phrases below is followed by a list of numbered words or phrases. MATCH the lettered word or phrase most closely associated with the numbered word or phrase.

Questions 9 through 13

A. venipuncture (depending on location of the collection area) has 4 to 10 units

B. rental space, administrative costs, cost of utilities

C. ratio of hours worked per CAP hour

D. change in proportion to the volume of work (e.g., supplies)

E. a charge for blood collection is made

9. Productivity index
10. CAP workload units
11. Budgetary indirect costs
12. Revenue
13. Variable cost

Questions 14 through 18

A. the first step in developing a formal phlebotomy education program

B. the second step in developing a formal phlebotomy education program

C. the third step in developing a formal phlebotomy education program

D. the fourth step in developing a formal phlebotomy education program

E. the fifth step in developing a formal phlebotomy education program

14. Requires a literature review of standards and guidelines for phlebotomy instruction as well as a review of other types of phlebotomy education programs

15. Review the verification of need and submit a preliminary proposal for a formal education program to the administration

16. Begins the development of a course syllabus

17. Develop a statement of need and identification of goals

18. Identification of educational resources

DIRECTIONS: Indicate whether each statement is TRUE or FALSE.

19. **True/False:** Table 10–1 is an example of the indirect costs of collecting a blood glucose specimen.

TABLE 10–1.

Labor (6 min/collection @ $4.50/h + $0.90 FICA, etc.)	$0.54
Collection tube	0.17
Needle	0.15
Alcohol swab	0.01
Tray ($15.00 depreciated over 5 years)	< 0.01
Requisition slip	0.05
Tourniquet ($0.12 @ 800 collections/tourniquet)	0.01
Gauze squares	0.04
Bandage, adhesive	0.04
Total	$1.02

20. **True/False:** One of the criteria for selecting students for most phlebotomy training programs is a high school diploma or General Educational Development (GED) test certification.

21. **True/False:** Graduates of a formal phlebotomy education program are eligible to take the phlebotomy examinations administered by NCA and ASCP Board of Registry.

22. **True/False:** The ultimate goal of a phlebotomy education program is to increase the time a medical technologist can work at the laboratory bench.

23. **True/False:** Employee benefits, such as group health insurance and FICA, usually are between 15% and 30% of an employee's salary.

24. **True/False:** For zero base budgeting, the phlebotomy supervisor reviews the current phlebotomy budget and adjusts the line item allocations for the next budget cycle.

25. **True/False:** The CAP unit is described as "one minute of technical, clinical and aide time" for each procedure.

DIRECTIONS: For each of the questions or incomplete statements below, ONE or MORE of the numbered responses are correct. In each case select

    A. if only 1, 2, and 3 are correct
    B. if only 1 and 3 are correct
    C. if only 2 and 4 are correct
    D. if only 4 is correct
    E. if all are correct

26. Which of the following should be included in a phlebotomy course syllabus?

    (1) class schedule
    (2) purpose of course
    (3) course objectives
    (4) instructor/faculty/institution

27. The following item(s) need to be considered in the preparation of a budget for phlebotomy

    (1) volume of patients' specimens
    (2) human hours required and the skills
    (3) equipment
    (4) supplies for the hematology analyzer

28. Which of the following item(s) should be maintained on each piece of equipment in the phlebotomy unit?

    (1) institutional identification tag number
    (2) location

(3) name
(4) color

29. The phlebotomy competencies achieved during the operation phase of the teaching process can be tested by

(1) homework questions
(2) a written quiz
(3) an essay examination
(4) clinically supervised bedside instruction

30. Which of the following is/are considered personal qualities expected of a phlebotomist?

(1) neat appearance
(2) confidence
(3) courteousness
(4) good looking

31. The category/categories in which quality control plays a part in the total quality assurance in the clinical laboratory is/are

(1) patient preparation
(2) specimen collection
(3) transportation, handling, and processing of specimens
(4) patient referral

DIRECTIONS: Each group of lettered words or phrases below is followed by a list of numbered words or phrases. MATCH the lettered word or phrase most closely associated with the numbered word or phrase.

Questions 32 through 36

A. preparation teaching phase
B. familiarization teaching phase
C. observation teaching phase
D. manipulation teaching phase
E. operation teaching phase

32. Role playing and practical examinations for student to demonstrate technical competence

33. Oral quiz, homework questions, written quiz

34. Clinically supervised bedside instruction according to checklist of tasks to master techniques in clinical setting

35. Oral quiz, student teaching instructor approach

36. Oral quiz, homework questions, and written quiz after seeing instructor demonstrations

Questions 37 through 39

A. testing for cognitive domain
B. testing of psychomotor domain
C. testing of affective domain

37. Role playing to demonstrate attitudes
38. Written examination to demonstrate knowledge, theory, and problem-solving skills
39. Practical examination to demonstrate phlebotomy skill

Answers and Explanations

1. **B.** To plan the implementation of a phlebotomy unit, the goals and mission of the hospital, agency, clinic, or company must be considered first.

   Garza D, Becan-McBride K. Phlebotomy Handbook. E. Norwalk, CT: Appleton & Lange; 1989:257.

2. **B.** The medical specialties of the physicians (e.g., pediatrics, oncology, geriatrics, obstetrics) indicate to some extent the types of phlebotomy supplies and equipment that are needed in the specimen collection unit.

   Garza and Becan-McBride, p 259.

3. **D.** Typically, the forecast budget has been used in budget preparation for the specimen collection area and other areas of the clinical laboratory.

   Garza and Becan-McBride, p 266.

4. **C.** Space, utilities, and administration do not necessarily fluctuate with a change in workload and, thus, usually are referred to as fixed costs in a budget.

   Garza and Becan-McBride, p 266.

5. **B.** Monitoring the resources and performance of a phlebotomy unit is a management activity that points to adjustments needed in budgeting, planning, and organizing.

   Garza and Becan-McBride, p 269.

6. **C.** The participative type or style of concern for people and production (Blake and Mouton) generally is agreed to be the best leadership approach.

   Garza and Becan-McBride, p 263.

7. **D.** In phlebotomy and other health care management activities, FTE stands for full-time employee.
    Garza and Becan-McBride, p 261.

8. **C.** The most important resource in accomplishing the objectives of the phlebotomy unit are the phlebotomists.
    Garza and Becan-McBride, p 264.

9. **C.** A productivity index may be obtained for the laboratory budget by calculating the ratio of hours worked per CAP hour.
    Garza and Becan-McBride, p 267.

10. **A.** Venipuncture (depending on location of the collection area) has been assigned 4 to 10 CAP workload units.
    Garza and Becan-McBride, p 268.

11. **B.** Budgetary indirect costs consist of the rental space, laboratory and institutional administrative costs, maintenance and janitorial service, and utilities.
    Garza and Becan-McBride, p 266.

12. **E.** The charge, or additional money generated by blood collection, is revenue.
    Garza and Becan-McBride, pp 266–267.

13. **D.** The variable costs, which include supplies, change in proportion to the volume of work.
    Garza and Becan-McBride, p 266.

14. **D.** The fourth step in developing a formal phlebotomy educational program requires a literature review of standards and guidelines for phlebotomy instruction as well as a review of other types of phlebotomy education programs.
    Garza and Becan-McBride, p 272.

15. **B.** The second step in developing a formal phlebotomy education program involves reviewing the verification of need and submitting a preliminary proposal for a formal education program to the administration.
    Garza and Becan-McBride, p 272.

16. **E.** The fifth step in developing a formal phlebotomy education program begins the development of a course syllabus.
    Garza and Becan-McBride, p 272.

17. **A.** The first step in developing a formal phlebotomy education program involves developing a statement of need and identification of goals.
    Garza and Becan-McBride, p 271.

18. **C.** The third step in developing a formal phlebotomy education program involves identification of educational resources.
    Garza and Becan-McBride, p 272.

19. **FALSE.** Table 10–1 is an example of the direct costs of collecting a blood glucose specimen.
    Garza and Becan-McBride, pp 266–269.

20. **TRUE.** One of the criteria to select students for most phlebotomy training programs is a high school diploma or General Education Development (GED) test certification.
    Garza and Becan-McBride, p 275.

21. **TRUE.** Graduates of a formal phlebotomy education program are eligible to take the phlebotomy examinations administered by NCA and ASCP Board of Registry.
    Garza and Becan-McBride, p 277; ASCP Board of Registry Examination Newsletter, May 1989.

22. **FALSE.** The ultimate goal of a phlebotomy education program is to increase quality health care to the patient.
    Garza and Becan-McBride, p 271.

23. **TRUE.** Employee benefits, such as group health insurance and FICA, usually are between 15% and 30% of an employee's salary.
    Garza and Becan-McBride, p 268.

24. **FALSE.** For zero base budgeting, the budget is one in which all items are justified anew as if no previous budget existed.
    Garza and Becan-McBride, p 266.

25. **TRUE.** The CAP unit is described as "one minute of technical, clinical and aide time" for each procedure.
    Garza and Becan-McBride, p 267.

26. **E.** A phlebotomy course syllabus needs to include the class schedule, purpose of course, course objectives, and instructor/faculty/institution.
    Garza and Becan-McBride, p 272.

27. **A.** The items to be considered in the preparation of a budget for phlebotomy include (1) volume of patients' specimens, (2) human hours required and the skills, and (3) equipment.
    Garza and Becan-McBride, p 267.

28. **A.** A list of each piece of equipment by name, institutional identification tag number, and location should be maintained by the phlebotomy supervisor, and a copy should be given to the laboratory administration.
    Garza and Becan-McBride, p 269.

29. **D.** The phlebotomy competencies achieved during the operation phase of teaching methods can be tested by clinically supervised bedside instruction according to a checklist of tasks to master techniques in the clinical setting.

    Garza and Becan-McBride, p 278; Golden TH. A college course for phlebotomists. MLO 1981.

30. **A.** The personal qualities expected of a phlebotomist are (1) neat appearance, (2) confidence, (3) concern for patient, (4) courteousness, and (5) adherence to rules of conduct of the department.

    Garza and Becan-McBride, p 261.

31. **A.** The categories in which quality control plays a part in the total quality assurance in the clinical laboratory are (1) patient preparation, (2) specimen collection, and (3) the transportation, handling, and processing of specimens.

    Garza and Becan-McBride, p 262.

32. **D.** For the manipulation teaching phase, role playing and practical examinations are used to demonstrate the student's technical competence.

    Garza and Becan-McBride, p 278.

33. **A.** For the preparation teaching phase, oral quizzes, homework questions, and written quizzes are used to test the student's competency level.

    Garza and Becan-McBride, p 277.

34. **E.** For the operation teaching phase, the student's competency is tested by using clinically supervised bedside instruction according to a checklist of tasks to master techniques in the clinical setting.

    Garza and Becan-McBride, p 278.

35. **C.** For the observation teaching phase, the student's competency level is tested by using oral quizzes and the student teaching instructor approach.

    Garza and Becan-McBride, p 277.

36. **B.** For the familiarization teaching phase, the student's competency level is tested by oral quizzes, homework questions, and written quizzes after seeing instructor demonstrations.

    Garza and Becan-McBride, p 277.

37. **C.** For the affective domain, role playing is used frequently to demonstrate the student's attitudes.

    Garza and Becan-McBride, p 278.

38. **A.** For the cognitive domain, written examinations are used to demonstrate knowledge, theory, and problem-solving skills of the student.
     Garza and Becan-McBride, p 278.

39. **B.** For the psychomotor domain, practical examinations are used to demonstrate phlebotomy skills and techniques.
     Garza and Becan-McBride, p 279.

Basic Requests in English, Spanish, French, and Vietnamese

Questions

DIRECTIONS: The following group of lettered words or phrases is followed by a list of numbered words or phrases. MATCH the lettered word or phrase most closely associated with the numbered word or phrase.

Questions 1 through 10

A. Buenos dias
B. Buenas noches
C. Necesito sacar le sangre
D. Ya tomo el desayuno?
E. Como se llama?
F. No debe de comer
G. Duele un poquito
H. Necesito picarle su dedo
I. Señor/Señorita
J. Favor de cerrar el puño

1. Good night
2. I need to stick your finger
3. Good day
4. What is your name?
5. I need to take a blood sample
6. Please make a fist
7. Mister/Miss
8. Have you had breakfast?
9. It hurts a little
10. You should not eat

Answers

1. **B.**

   Garza D, Becan-McBride K. Phlebotomy Handbook. E. Norwalk, CT: Appleton & Lange; 1989:285–287.

2. **H.**

   Garza and Becan-McBride, pp 285–287.

3. **A.**

    Garza and Becan-McBride, pp 285–287.

4. **E.**

    Garza and Becan-McBride, pp 285–287.

5. **C.**

    Garza and Becan-McBride, pp 285–287.

6. **J.**

    Garza and Becan-McBride, pp 285–287.

7. **I.**

    Garza and Becan-McBride, pp 285–287.

8. **D.**

    Garza and Becan-McBride, pp 285–287.

9. **G.**

    Garza and Becan-McBride, pp 285–287.

10. **F.**

    Garza and Becan-McBride, pp 285–287.

Units of Measurement

Questions

DIRECTIONS: Each lettered abbreviation or symbol below is followed by a list of numbered words or phrases. MATCH the lettered abbreviation or symbol with the appropriate numbered word or phrase.

Questions 1 through 10

A.	°C	**1.**	Quantity not sufficient
B.	kg	**2.**	Greater than or equal to
C.	QNS	**3.**	Degrees Kelvin—unit of temperature
D.	≤	**4.**	Less than or equal to
E.	mm³	**5.**	Low-power field on a microscope
F.	≥	**6.**	Liter
G.	L	**7.**	Degrees Celsius—unit of temperature
H.	°K	**8.**	Kilogram
I.	lpf	**9.**	Degrees Fahrenheit—unit of temperature
J.	°F	**10.**	Cubic millimeter

Answers

1. **C.**

   Garza D, Becan-McBride K. Phlebotomy Handbook. E. Norwalk, CT: Appleton & Lange; 1989:289–290.

2. **F.**

   Garza and Becan-McBride, pp 289–290.

3. **H.**

   Garza and Becan-McBride, pp 289–290.

4. **D.**

   Garza and Becan-McBride, pp 289–290.

5. **I.**

   Garza and Becan-McBride, pp 289–290.

6. **G.**

   Garza and Becan-McBride, pp 289–290.

7. **A.**

   Garza and Becan-McBride, pp 289–290.

8. **B.**

   Garza and Becan-McBride, pp 289–290.

9. **J.**

   Garza and Becan-McBride, pp 289–290.

10. **E.**

    Garza and Becan-McBride, pp 289–290.

Metric Conversion Chart

Questions

DIRECTIONS: Each lettered measurement below is followed by a list of numbered units. MATCH the lettered measurement with the appropriate numbered unit.

Questions 1 through 5

A. 39.37 inches	**1.** One kilogram
B. 3.78 liters	**2.** One foot
C. 2.54 centimeters	**3.** One meter
D. 2.2 pounds	**4.** One gallon
E. 30.48 centimeters	**5.** One inch

Answers

1. **D.**

   Garza D, Becan-McBride K. Phlebotomy Handbook. *E. Norwalk, CT: Appleton & Lange; 1989:291.*

2. **E.**

   Garza and Becan-McBride, p 291.

3. **A.**

   Garza and Becan-McBride, p 291.

4. **B.**

   Garza and Becan-McBride, p 291.

5. **C.**

   Garza and Becan-McBride, p 291.

Formulas and Calculations

Questions

DIRECTIONS: Each lettered word or phrase below is followed by a list of numbered words or phrases. MATCH the lettered word or phrase with the appropriate numbered word or phrase.

Questions 1 through 5

A. Sp g	**1.** Specific gravity
B. volt	**2.** Frequency
C. square meter	**3.** Area
D. Hertz	**4.** Hematologic value
E. MCV	**5.** Electrical potential

Answers

1. **A.**

   Garza D, Becan-McBride K. Phlebotomy Handbook. *E. Norwalk, CT: Appleton & Lange; 1989:293–295.*

2. **D.**

   Garza and Becan-McBride, pp 293–295.

3. **C.**

   Garza and Becan-McBride, pp 293–295.

4. **E.**

   Garza and Becan-McBride, pp 293–295.

5. **B.**

   Garza and Becan-McBride, pp 293–295.

Medical Terminology

Questions

DIRECTIONS: The lettered abbreviations are commonly used for laboratory tests. MATCH the lettered abbreviation with the appropriate numbered word or phrase.

A.	VMA	1.	Tuberculosis
B.	LDH	2.	Epstein-Barr virus
C.	PTT	3.	High density lipoprotein
D.	RA	4.	Electrolytes
E.	PKU	5.	Arterial blood gases
F.	VLDL	6.	Prothrombin time
G.	O & P	7.	Glucose-6-phosphatase dehydrogenase
H.	IgA	8.	Luteinizing hormone
I.	RPR	9.	Rheumatoid arthritis
J.	ABG	10.	White blood cell
K.	LH	11.	Vanillylmandelic acid
L.	TB	12.	Ova and parasites
M.	EBV	13.	Lactic dehydrogenase
N.	Mg	14.	Phenylketonuria
O.	PT	15.	Erythrocyte sedimentation rate
P.	WBC	16.	Rapid plasma reagin (for syphilis)
Q.	HDL	17.	Partial thromboplastin time
R.	lytes	18.	Magnesium
S.	G-6-P-D	19.	Immunoglobulin A
T.	ESR	20.	Very low density lipoprotein

DIRECTIONS: The lettered medical prefixes, suffixes, or abbreviations describe certain conditions or locations on the human body. MATCH the lettered items with the appropriate numbered medical term.

A. thrombo-	21. Gastrointestinal
B. SIDS	22. Brain
C. proximal	23. Inflammation
D. distal	24. Large
E. carcino-	25. Blueness
F. pseudo-	26. Breaking down
G. macro	27. Heart
H. -ology	28. Mouth
I. AIDS	29. Ear, nose, throat
J. DOA	30. Near the body trunk
K. GI	31. Intravenous
L. -lysis	32. Small
M. cerebro-	33. Cancer
N. IV	34. Away from body trunk
O. os	35. Clot
P. -itis	36. Acquired immunodeficiency syndrome
Q. cyano-	37. Sudden infant death syndrome
R. ENT	38. The study of
S. micro-	39. False
T. cardio-	40. Dead on arrival

DIRECTIONS: Indicate whether each statement is TRUE or FALSE.

41. **True/False:** STAT means "immediately" or "now."
42. **True/False:** Segos is another term for neutrophils.
43. **True/False:** Septic usually refers to something sterile.
44. **True/False:** T & S frequently indicates a procedure prior to blood transfusion.
45. **True/False:** The X chromosome is the female chromosome.
46. **True/False:** Na and K are chemical symbols for sodium and potassium, respectively.
47. **True/False:** Myocardium is the heart muscle.
48. **True/False:** The chemical symbol NaCl means sodium hydroxide.
49. **True/False:** Reference to an electrolyte battery usually means Na, Cl, K, bicarbonate.
50. **True/False:** The terms crit and Hct frequently are used for hematocrit.
51. **True/False:** Pediatrics is the study of the foot bones and muscles.
52. **True/False:** C & S usually refers to a microbiologic culture and antibiotic sensitivity test.
53. **True/False:** Water is chemically abbreviated as HO_2.
54. **True/False:** Anemia can be detected by routine hematology laboratory tests.
55. **True/False:** Toxicology refers to the study of drugs and poisons.

Answers

1. **L.**

   Garza D, Becan-McBride K. Phlebotomy Handbook. *E. Norwalk, CT: Appleton & Lange; 1989:297–308.*

2. **M.**

   Garza and Becan-McBride, pp 297–308.

3. **Q.**

   Garza and Becan-McBride, pp 297–308.

4. **R.**

   Garza and Becan-McBride, pp 297–308.

5. **J.**

   Garza and Becan-McBride, pp 297–308.

6. **O.**

   Garza and Becan-McBride, pp 297–308.

7. **S.**

   Garza and Becan-McBride, pp 297–308.

8. **K.**

   Garza and Becan-McBride, pp 297–308.

9. **D.**

   Garza and Becan-McBride, pp 297–308.

10. **P.**

    Garza and Becan-McBride, pp 297–308.

11. **A.**

    Garza and Becan-McBride, pp 297–308.

12. **G.**

    Garza and Becan-McBride, pp 297–308.

13. **B.**

    Garza and Becan-McBride, pp 297–308.

14. **E.**

    Garza and Becan-McBride, pp 297–308.

15. **T.**

    Garza and Becan-McBride, pp 297–308.

16. **I.**

    Garza and Becan-McBride, pp 297–308.

17. **C.**
    Garza and Becan-McBride, pp 297–308.

18. **N.**
    Garza and Becan-McBride, pp 297–308.

19. **H.**
    Garza and Becan-McBride, pp 297–308.

20. **F.**
    Garza and Becan-McBride, pp 297–308.

21. **K.**
    Garza and Becan-McBride, pp 297–308.

22. **M.**
    Garza and Becan-McBride, pp 297–308.

23. **P.**
    Garza and Becan-McBride, pp 297–308.

24. **G.**
    Garza and Becan-McBride, pp 297–308.

25. **Q.**
    Garza and Becan-McBride, pp 297–308.

26. **L.**
    Garza and Becan-McBride, pp 297–308.

27. **T.**
    Garza and Becan-McBride, pp 297–308.

28. **O.**
    Garza and Becan-McBride, pp 297–308.

29. **R.**
    Garza and Becan-McBride, pp 297–308.

30. **C.**
    Garza and Becan-McBride, pp 297–308.

31. **N.**
    Garza and Becan-McBride, pp 297–308.

32. **S.**
    Garza and Becan-McBride, pp 297–308.

33. **E.**
    Garza and Becan-McBride, pp 297–308.

34. **D.**
    Garza and Becan-McBride, pp 297–308.

35. **A.**
Garza and Becan-McBride, pp 297–308.

36. **I.**
Garza and Becan-McBride, pp 297–308.

37. **B.**
Garza and Becan-McBride, pp 297–308.

38. **H.**
Garza and Becan-McBride, pp 297–308.

39. **F.**
Garza and Becan-McBride, pp 297–308.

40. **J.**
Garza and Becan-McBride, pp 297–308.

41. **TRUE.**
Garza and Becan-McBride, pp 297–308.

42. **FALSE.**
Garza and Becan-McBride, pp 297–308.

43. **FALSE.**
Garza and Becan-McBride, pp 297–308.

44. **TRUE.**
Garza and Becan-McBride, pp 297–308.

45. **TRUE.**
Garza and Becan-McBride, pp 297–308.

46. **TRUE.**
Garza and Becan-McBride, pp 297–308.

47. **TRUE.**
Garza and Becan-McBride, pp 297–308.

48. **FALSE.**
Garza and Becan-McBride, pp 297–308.

49. **TRUE.**
Garza and Becan-McBride, pp 297–308.

50. **TRUE.**
Garza and Becan-McBride, pp 297–308.

51. **FALSE.**
Garza and Becan-McBride, pp 297–308.